Coincidence or Crisis?

Prescription medicine counterfeiting

Jonathan Harper, Julian Morris, Graham Satchwell, Philip Stevens, David Taylor, Michael Tremblay

Foreword by Mark E. Souder
Introduction by Bill Newton Dunn

Edited by Peter J. Pitts

CENTRE FOR THE NEW EUROPE

CMPI
Center for Medicine in the Public Interest

STOCKHOLM NETWORK

First published in Great Britain in 2006 by
The Stockholm Network
35 Britannia Row
London N1 8QH
www.stockholm-network.org

in association with Profile Books Ltd

Reprinted in 2007

The Stockholm Network is Europe's only dedicated service organisation for market-oriented think tanks and thinkers

A CIP catalogue record for this book is available from the British Library.

ISBN-10: 0-9547663-8-5
ISBN-13: 978-0-9547663-8-2

Designed by Sue Lamble
Typeset in Stone Serif by MacGuru Ltd
info@macguru.org.uk

Printed and bound in Great Britain by Hobbs the Printers

Coincidence or Crisis?

Prescription medicine counterfeiting

The Stockholm Network

The Stockholm Network is Europe's leading pan-European think tank and market-oriented network. A one-stop shop for organisations seeking to work with Europe's brightest policy-makers and thinkers, our unique network of over 120 market-oriented think tanks in Europe and farther afield provides unparalleled access to the best European policy thinking, the opportunity to lead debates, to change the climate of ideas in Europe, and to meet the key players in shaping the policy debates of tomorrow.

Contents

About the contributors

Dr Jonathan Harper, BSc (Hons), MB ChB, MBA (LBS) is a pharmaceutical and health sector consultant with extensive experience in central and eastern Europe. He was the author of the Council of Europe's 2006 counterfeit medicines report (jrharper@axelero.hu).

Julian Morris, MA (Edin), MSc (London), MPhil (Cantab), Grad Dip. Law (Westminster), is executive director of International Policy Network, a London-based development charity, and a visiting professor at the University of Buckingham's Department of International Studies.

Bill Newton Dunn, MA (Cantab), MBA (INSEAD), is Liberal Democrat MEP for the East Midlands. He is a full member of the Internal Market and Consumer Protection Committee of the Parliament and an associate member of the Justice and Home Affairs Committee. He is the Liberal Democrat whip in the Parliament.

Peter J. Pitts is director of the Center for Medicine in the Public Interest and Senior Vice-President for Global Health Affairs at

Manning Selvage & Lee. From 2002 to 2004 he was Associate Commissioner for External Relations at the US Food and Drug Administration.

Graham Satchwell, LL.B (Hons), FRSA, is a British security expert. A former detective superintendent, Graham led successful criminal and civil investigations of counterfeit brand-name goods, including pharmaceuticals, throughout Europe, Asia and the developing world. Graham runs a specialist anti-conterfeiting company, ProcoSolutions.com, chairs the UK government Patent Office Brands Group, and consults for several global corporations.

Mark E. Souder is a US Congressman from Indiana's 3rd District and is chairman of the Subcommittee on Criminal Justice, Drug Policy and Human Resources of the Government Reform Committee in the US House of Representatives.

Philip Stevens is Health Programme Director at the London-based International Policy Network.

David Taylor is Professor of Pharmaceutical and Public Health Policy at the University of London School of Pharmacy and recently a member of the Advisory Group on the Reform of the NHS Pharmaceutical Services (david.taylor@pharmacy.ac.uk).

Dr Michael Tremblay is a former adviser to the Council of Europe and the government of Great Britain, who currently runs Tremblay Consulting (www.tremblay-consulting.biz).

Preface

21st-century international drug terrorism

Peter J. Pitts

This is a book about false profits, the frightening and dangerous growth in international prescription drug counterfeiting.

When asked why he robbed banks, Willy Sutton, the American Depression-era criminal, replied, 'Because that's where the money is.' And, as former FDA Commissioner Mark McClellan used to say, if Sutton were alive today he'd be selling counterfeit prescription drugs.

The bad news is that international prescription drug counterfeiting is on the rise.

Watching the international news wires is to witness the growth of this insidious criminal epidemic. From China we learn of eleven Chinese nationals and one American arrested in a counterfeit medicine scheme that spanned eleven countries, 440,000 bogus pills and US$4.3 million. The drugs being peddled were Lipitor, Viagra, Cialis and Levitra. The nations involved were the USA, Great Britain, Switzerland and Israel.

From Hamilton, Ontario, we learn of a registered pharmacist charged with selling counterfeit Norvasc. The regional coroner in Hamilton is currently investigating the deaths of five people who filled prescriptions for Norvasc at this pharmacy. All five died of a heart attack or stroke. From the US Attorney's Office we learn of the indictment of eighteen people alleged to have taken part in a multimillion-dollar international conspiracy to smuggle cigarettes and counterfeit Viagra to raise money for the Middle East terrorist group Hezbollah.

'The enterprise operated from Lebanon, Canada, Brazil, Paraguay, China, North Carolina, Florida and the Dearborn, Michigan area, perpetrating crimes in the states of Michigan, California, Florida, Georgia, Illinois, North Carolina and West Virginia (and points in between),' the indictment alleges.

The EU recently went on the record (again) with its concerns about the rise of counterfeit drugs in Europe, and Canadian authorities reported that they have made arrests in their ongoing 'Project Piranha', seizing a Hell's Angels gang's supply of marijuana, hashish – and counterfeit prescription drugs.

When, two years ago, the FDA stated publicly that counterfeit drug schemes were being used to fund global terrorist organisations, certain governors and members of Congress accused the agency of 'being in the pocket of Big Pharma'. Well, they are strangely silent today. And the recent news that the government of North Korea is in the business of manufacturing and selling counterfeit prescription drugs puts this problem into dramatic perspective – it is nothing short of international healthcare terrorism.

Coincidence or crisis?

In the not-too-recent past many blustering elected officials on both sides of the Atlantic regularly called the threat of counterfeit prescription medicines a 'ploy' by the pharmaceutical industry. Not any more. Today it's a question of seeing and believing.

To respond to this emerging threat, the FDA formed a Counterfeit Drug Task Force in July 2003. As an FDA Associate Commissioner, I was proud to serve as a member of that task force. We received extensive comment from security experts, federal and state law enforcement officials, technology developers, manufacturers, wholesalers, retailers, consumer groups and the general public on a very broad range of ideas for deterring counterfeiters.

Those comments reinforced the need for the FDA to take action in multiple areas to create a comprehensive system of modern protections against counterfeit drugs.

At the FDA we discussed those ideas, and developed a framework for a 21st-century pharmaceutical supply chain that would be more secure against modern counterfeit threats.

The specific approach to assuring that Americans are protected from counterfeit drugs includes the following eight elements:

1. Implementation of new technologies to better protect our drug supply.
2. Adoption of electronic track and trace technology.
3. Adoption and enforcement of strong, proven anti-counterfeiting laws and regulations by individual US states.
4. Increased criminal penalties to deter counterfeiting and more adequately punish those convicted.
5. Adoption of secure business practices by all participants in the drug supply chain.

6 Development of a system that helps ensure effective reporting of counterfeit drugs to the FDA and which strengthens the agency's rapid response to such reports.

7 Education of consumers and health professionals about the risks of counterfeit drugs and how to protect against them.

8 Collaboration with foreign stakeholders to develop strategies to deter and detect counterfeit drugs globally.

Counterfeit drugs are a global challenge to all nations, and criminal counterfeiting operations are increasingly operating across national borders. The FDA intends to work with the WHO, Interpol and other international public health and law enforcement organisations to develop and implement worldwide strategies to combat counterfeit drugs. To that end, the February 2006 'Conclusions and Recommendations of the WHO International Conference on Combating Counterfeit Medicines' are a very important next step in the harmonisation of resolve and resources in the war against international prescription drug counterfeiting:

> The participants of the WHO International Conference 'Combating Counterfeit Drugs: Building Effective International Collaboration', gathered in Rome on 18 February 2006
>
> DECLARE
>
> 1 Counterfeiting medicines, including the entire range of activities from manufacturing to providing them to patients, is a vile and serious criminal offence that puts human lives at risk and undermines the credibility of health systems.

2 Because of its direct impact on health, counterfeiting medicines should be combated and punished accordingly.

3 Combating counterfeit medicines requires the coordinated effort of all the different public and private stakeholders that are affected and are competent for addressing the different aspects of the problem.

4 Counterfeiting medicines is widespread and has escalated to such an extent that effective coordination and cooperation at the international level are necessary for regional and national strategies to be more effective.

5 National, regional and international strategies aimed at combating counterfeit medicines should be based on:

a) Political will, adequate legal framework, and implementation commensurate to the impact of this type of counterfeiting on public health and providing the necessary tools for a coordinated and effective law enforcement,

b) Inter-sectoral coordination based on written procedures, clearly defined roles, adequate resources, and effective administrative and operational tools,

c) Creating an awareness about the severity of the problem among all stakeholders and providing information to all levels of the health system and the public,

d) Development of technical competence and skills in all required areas,

- e) Appropriate mechanisms for ensuring vigilance and input from healthcare professionals and the public.

6 The WHO should lead the establishment of an International Medical Products Anti-Counterfeiting Taskforce (IMPACT) of governmental, non-governmental and international institutions aimed at:

- a) Raising awareness among international organizations and other stakeholders at the international level in order to improve cooperation in combating counterfeit medicines, taking into account its global dimensions
- b) Raising awareness among national authorities and decision-makers and calling for effective legislative measures in order to combat counterfeit medicines
- c) Establishing effective exchange of information and providing assistance on specific issues that concern combating counterfeit medicines
- d) Developing technical and administrative tools to support the establishment or strengthening of international, regional and national strategies
- e) Encouraging coordination among different anti-counterfeiting initiatives.

The IMPACT will function on the basis of existing structures/institutions and will in the long term explore further mechanisms, including an international convention, for strengthening international action against counterfeit medicines.

One of the most serious impediments to an allied transatlantic war against prescription drug counterfeiters is parallel trade. Last year 140 million individual drug packages were parallel-imported throughout the European Union – and a wholesaler repackaged each and every one.

This means that, literally, parallel traders open 140 million packets of drugs, remove their contents and repackage them. But these parallel profiteers are in the moneymaking business, not the safety business. And mistakes happen. For example, new labels incorrectly state the dosage strength; a new label says the box contains tablets, but inside are capsules; the expiration date and batch numbers on the medicine boxes don't match the actual batch and dates of expiration of the medicines inside; and patient information materials are often in the wrong language or are out of date.

This means that a prescription drug that comes from a British chemist, purchased by an unknowing American consumer from a Canadian Internet pharmacy, could in fact come from European Union nations such as Greece, Latvia, Poland, Malta, Cyprus or Estonia. In fact, parallel-traded medicines account for about 20% (one in five) of all prescriptions filled by British pharmacies. In the EU there is no requirement to record the batch numbers of parallel-imported medicines, so if a batch of medicines originally intended for sale in Greece is recalled, tracing where the entire batch has gone (for example, from Athens to London through Canada to Indianapolis) is impossible. Caveat emptor is bad healthcare practice and even worse healthcare policy. Safety cannot be compromised, even if the truth is inconvenient.

More dangerous even than the lack of more robust quality

control is the opening such practices provide to criminal counterfeiters to integrate their phoney products into the legitimate supply chains in both Europe and North America. The World Health Organisation estimates that between 8 and 10% of the global medicine supply chain is counterfeit – rising to 25% or higher in some countries. The largest counterfeit market with close proximity to the EU free trade zone is Russia, where the generally accepted estimate is that 12% of drugs are counterfeit. Now that the Baltic nations of Latvia, Lithuania and Estonia have joined the European Union, the WHO has warned that an increase in the risks of counterfeits entering the EU supply chain is 'obvious'. Facts are stubborn things.

There's a Japanese proverb that bears repeating – 'Don't fix the blame. Fix the problem'.

On 20 September 2005, the Center for Medicine in the Public Interest held a one-day conference on the dangers of international prescription drug counterfeiting in Washington, DC, and on 15 February 2006 a similar event was held (in collaboration with the Centre for the New Europe) in Brussels. The following chapters are by the presenters at these two conferences. They offer creative, timely and, most importantly, practical and functional solutions to this crucial global public health crisis.

We are also pleased to offer two introductory pieces from either side of the Atlantic by two respected public figures: a foreword by the Honorable Mark Souder, United States Congressman, and an introduction by the Honourable Bill Newton Dunn, Member of the European Parliament.

Let us move forward with the words of former Canadian prime minister Pierre Trudeau, who said, '*Renversons les totems, casser les taboux*. Let us overthrow the totems, break the taboos. Or better yet, let us consider them cancelled. Coldly, let us be intelligent.'

Foreword

Mark E. Souder

The important theme of this timely compilation is that the manufacturing and selling of fake prescription drugs is a serious – even deadly – public threat, and a fast-growing, international problem that demands attention.

The current estimate by the World Health Organisation that 10% of global pharmaceutical commerce this year will be counterfeit is startling. That this number is expected to double by the year 2010, as international criminal organisations become more sophisticated, is a clarion call for international action.

Counterfeit drug commerce affects every country, every class of people, through all kinds of commercial transactions. It is not limited to Internet purchases and flea markets, but touches even major distributors providing drugs to large pharmaceutical chains. Everyone is vulnerable to this nefarious business.

I have chaired congressional hearings in the United States House of Representatives that have focused on the critical problem of counterfeit drugs. I firmly believe this is an issue that must be challenged aggressively, because, unlike other forms of counterfeit and fraud, fake pharmaceuticals put people's lives at stake. No government can afford to wait until there is a catastrophic failure in the system before confronting the problems that facilitate counterfeit pharmaceutical commerce.

In the past five years, the US drug market has experienced a massive increase in counterfeit and sub-standard pharmaceuticals. In 2000, seizures of fake pharmaceuticals accounted for fewer than an estimated 100,000 doses. But by 2004 it is estimated that more than 3 million fake medications were seized in the United States. Although Internet purchases account for a large proportion of counterfeit drugs (currently there are hundreds of sites that offer prescription drugs without a prescription or examination by a physician; and over 100,000 packages arrive daily in the USA from overseas pharmacies), the Internet is not the only source.

Typically, drug manufacturers exert no control over drug products beyond their loading docks. Drugs go through several middlemen before reaching a patient's hands, and are continually vulnerable to counterfeit practices each time. When such middlemen resell the drugs, they sometimes relabel them to reflect higher (and more valuable) doses, or substitute fake products for the legitimate goods. Diverters also breach the supply chain by introducing drugs that have been acquired by fraud or criminal theft.

This collection of essays takes a critical look at various gaps that allow for the proliferation of counterfeit pharmaceuticals, and offers substantive, cross-cutting approaches for confronting the counterfeit drug problem. Unique regional issues such as parallel trade, porous borders, regulatory enforcement and property rights are all taken up in this comprehensive look at a serious and growing global problem.

Counterfeit pharmaceuticals are a growing international

problem that will require governments to work together. Complacency is not an option when prevalence is increasing, and such drugs are killing people. Confronting the complexity of the problem makes plain that there are no easy answers, but this book is an essential starting point for understanding the scope of the problem, the vulnerabilities and the different layers of solutions that will be required by governments and industry.

Introduction

Bill Newton Dunn

This book is both important and timely. There is a steady – although still unmeasured – growth in all types of international organised crime. But whereas fake perfumes or fake jeans or pirated music may turn out to be a disappointment, fake pharmaceutical products are infinitely more serious – because they may damage the health of the consumer.

Europeans are failing to counter all these organised crimes. The basic problem is that the gangs cross open borders inside Europe with impunity. But all our police forces are national, and therefore cannot cross frontiers. What is 'hot' in one state seems of less importance next door.

There are no statistics to measure the growth of crime across Europe – because each of the 25 member states of the European Union collects its own figures in its own way. But my feeling is that crime is growing on all fronts because it is not being fought.

There is no European police force to fight the international gangs on their own terms. Both Interpol and Europol are located in Europe. Interpol in Lyon is a club, financed by policemen around the world, which acts as a worldwide information centre, and holds valuable databases. Europol in The Hague is the European Union's intelligence-gathering centre, which also holds databases, and is financed by the 25 national governments of the EU. But neither of the two organisations' staff have operational or arrest powers.

The criminal gangs are based, mostly, in eastern Europe or farther east. Often made up of ethnic families, they contain bright people who cannot find legitimate employment in their own country. They operate as tight, highly efficient but ruthless and cruel businesses which are quick to spot market opportunities. They traffic heroin from Afghanistan, cocaine from Colombia and ecstasy from Europe. They traffic illegal immigrants from Asia and Africa, women for prostitution, and children for paedophilia. They phish for people's identities over the Internet with the purpose of stealing their money. They counterfeit goods and currency. They violently steal luxury motor cars and, of course, they fake and traffic pharmaceuticals.

Why are European governments ineffective in fighting organised international crime? After all, the Home Office in London recently said that 'every kilo of heroin imported into the UK causes over 200 street crimes'. They know it would pay them handsome dividends.

The reason for their failure is nationalism, and their lack of trust of other Europeans. Each national government and parliament thinks it knows best. Each is reluctant to share information with others for the greater European good. When they share information, they are unwilling to authenticate it by revealing their sources. Meanwhile, the gangs cooperate internationally and remain unchallenged for too long.

Europe needs to create its own cross-border law enforcement agency with operational powers. The USA has its FBI. Europe has nothing. The gutter press would complain that 'foreigners in jackboots are now arresting our citizens at dead of night. Didn't we fight the Second World War to prevent this?' Instead of being afraid of such criticism, Europe's national leaders should look forward and provide leadership in solving our new problems, such as organised crime.

If they continue not to do so, the gangs will prosper and grow, and eat away at the fabric of our society. The stronger the gangs grow, the more difficult it will become to counter them, and the more our law-abiding societies will fray and crumble – leading, as is all too visible in many parts of the world, to failed states in Europe.

Acronyms used in the text

ADR	Adverse drug reaction
API	Active pharmaceutical ingredient (active substance)
BAPW	British Association of Pharmaceutical Wholesalers
BP	Bulk/intermediate pharmaceutical product
CEP	Certificate of Suitability of European Pharmacopoeia monographs
CM	Counterfeit medicine
CoA	Certificate of Analysis
CoE	Council of Europe
CoS	Certificate of Suitability
DMF	Drug Master File
EC	European Commission
FP	Finished medicinal product
FTA	Free trade agreement
GDP	Good Distribution Practice
GMP	Good Manufacturing Practice
GTDP	Good Trade and Distribution Practice
ICH	International Conference on Harmonisation of technical requirements for registration of pharmaceuticals for human use

LDC	Less developed country(ies)
IPR	Intellectual (industrial) property rights
MA	Marketing Authorisation
MAA	Marketing Authorisation Application
MAH	Marketing Authorisation Holder
PC	Pharmaceutical crime
PI	Parallel importation
RAS	Rapid Alert System
SPOC	Single point of contact
TRIPs	Trade-related aspects of intellectual property rights

1

Counterfeit medicines and pharmaceutical crime in Europe: 'invisibility, biohazard and system failure'

Findings and recommendations from the Council of Europe survey report

Jonathan Harper

Introduction

This chapter presents and discusses the medicines counterfeiting situation in Europe from the perspective of the Council of Europe (CoE) counterfeit medicines survey report entitled *Harmonised Provisions for Legislative and Administrative Procedures Applicable to Counterfeit Medicines in the Council of Europe Member States*, completed in early 2005 and published in January 2006 (Harper, 2006). The predominant themes behind counterfeit medicines (CM) and pharmaceutical crime (PC) that come out of the report are those of *invisibility, biohazard* and *system failure.* Furthermore, from the list of report topics presented in Box 1, it can be seen that the subject of counterfeit medicines is a complex one in terms of both causality and potential solutions.

Box 1 Council of Europe counterfeit medicine report topics

1. Definitions of 'counterfeit medicine' and 'pharmaceutical crime'
2. Epidemiology behind the CM phenomenon
3. The CM market (historical, current and future)
4. Impact of CM and PC on public health
5. Adequacy of pharmaceutical manufacturing regulation in the context of CM (API and FP, packaging, labelling)
6. CM trade and distribution (parallel trade, Internet pharmacy, regulation of pharmaceutical import/export/transit, unlicensed medicines, brokers, traders, legal and illegal (and non-regulated) distribution chain, FP security and traceability, organised crime, etc.)
7. Adequacy of systems to detect CM: authorities, customs, systems and procedures (who, what and how)
8. Intellectual property rights (with respect to CM/PC)
9. Legal and enforcement provisions/systems (including sanctions and penalties)
10. Cooperation/coordination (national and international authority/stakeholders)
11. Stakeholder CM problem perception (and impact on health system perception)
12. Perceived European system adequacy (for tackling CM/PC)
13. Professional training (authority and stakeholder CM detection and control)
14. Conclusions and recommendations (by survey respondents and report author)

Background to the Council of Europe counterfeit medicine survey and report

Based on its public health protection, anti-crime and societal governance mandate, in late 2003 the CoE identified the need for an initiative to look in detail at the counterfeit medicine and pharmaceutical crime situation in Europe and its impact on public health and the legitimate pharmaceutical economy.

Thus, between 2003 and 2004, the CoE conducted extensive surveys of (i) relevant national authorities responsible for health/pharmaceutical regulation, interior affairs/law enforcement, judicial/legal affairs, finance/tax/customs and economy/trade; (ii) stakeholders covering the pharmaceutical manufacturing and distribution chain (see Box 2). The information from these surveys forms the basis of the CoE report.

Definitions of counterfeit medicine, pharmaceutical crime and diversion

When the topic of counterfeit medicines is discussed, it is important first to have an accurate understanding of what exactly counterfeit medicines and pharmaceutical crime are. It is also important to have an understanding of what diversion is, as this practice is a part of pharmaceutical crime and also linked to medicines counterfeiting. These definitions are presented in Box 3 below.

The WHO states that counterfeit medicines are part of the broader phenomenon of sub-standard pharmaceuticals – medicines manufactured below established standards of safety, quality and efficacy. In the context of the CoE report and this

Box 2 Council of Europe surveys conducted

1 2003 CoE Member State Survey
(8 of 26 CoE member state ministries of health/drug regulatory authorities that are signatories to the Council of Europe Partial Agreement in the Social and Public Health Field)

2 2004 CoE Member State Authorities Survey
(13 of 26 member state signatories to the Council of Europe Partial Agreement in the Social and Public Health Field), including:

- ministries of health/drug regulatory authorities
- ministries for interior affairs/national police agencies
- ministries of justice (jurisdiction, prosecution, civil and penal procedures)
- ministries of finance/tax and customs agencies
- ministries of economy/trade

3 2004 CoE Intellectual Property Rights (IPR) and National Criminal Law Comparative Study
(survey of the 46 CoE member states)

4 2004 Stakeholder Survey
(30 companies represented by the following associations)

- Active pharmaceutical ingredient manufacturers: APIC (Active Pharmaceutical Ingredient Committee) and CEFIC (European Chemical Industry Council)

- Finished medicinal product manufacturers: EFPIA (European Federation of Pharmaceutical Industry Associations)
- Wholesalers: GIRP (Groupement International de la Repartition Pharmaceutique/European Association of Full-line Pharmaceutical Wholesalers)
- Veterinary products: IFAH (International Federation for Animal Health)

chapter, counterfeit medicine is meant in the sense of the WHO definition (WHO, 2006a), as this seems to be the most widely accepted definition which covers counterfeiting of the product itself and/or the packaging and labelling. Concerning pharmaceutical crime, there is no commonly accepted definition; items and conceptual points that should be considered under such a definition are presented below. A good definition of diversion is provided by Satchwell (2004).

The extent of the counterfeit medicine problem in Europe

Fundamental questions that need answering are whether counterfeit medicines are a real threat to public health and also to the legitimate pharmaceutical economy in Europe.

Do counterfeit medicines exist in Europe?

The evidence from the CoE survey report suggests that counterfeit medicines exist practically everywhere in Europe and

Box 3 Definitions of counterfeit medicine, pharmaceutical crime and diversion

WHO definition of counterfeit medicine (WHO, 2006a)

A product that is deliberately and fraudulently mislabelled with respect to identity and/or source. Counterfeiting can apply to both branded and generic products and counterfeit medicines may include products with the correct ingredients but fake packaging, with the wrong ingredients, without active ingredients or with insufficient active ingredients.

Items and conceptual points that should be considered in defining pharmaceutical crime include:

Pharmaceutical crime

- Incorporation of pharmaceutical crime under the definition heading of health crime (the latter relating to health risk and damage)
- Differentiation of medicines counterfeiting from other types of product counterfeiting by use of the concept of 'aggravated circumstances of counterfeiting and piracy'
- A formal classification of types of medicines counterfeiting that is linked to a scale of degree of regulatory violation and appropriate penalties
- Possession
- Intent
- Falsification (product, packaging, documentation)
- Fraud

- Intellectual property rights (IPR) – both for patented products and for IPR protection extension to authorised generics
- Unauthorised and illegal manufacturing, brokering, distribution and retailing
- Diversion (see below)
- Manufacturer, distributer and retailer tort

Diversion (Satchwell, 2004)
Diversion is the movement of branded goods across international markets, contrary to the wishes and legal rights of the brand owner. The word 'diversion' cannot be used for the unwanted (by the brand owner) movement of goods within the European Union, as it is legally a single market. Sometimes the word 'grey' is used to describe diverted products.

are not just confined to eastern Europe. First real evidence for the presence of counterfeit medicines on the European market appeared in *circa* 1998, and since then the number of cases reported has been steadily increasing (Harper, 2006).

Undoubtedly there is a large 'invisibility' factor that masks the real extent of the presence of counterfeit medicines in Europe. This is due to a number of reasons, not least of which are the very nature of medicinal products (counterfeit medicines are invariably harder to detect compared with other types of counterfeited products), the lack of a commonly agreed and employed definition of counterfeit medicines (if we do not know how to define something then it is difficult to record and estimate its presence) by European states, and a lack of awareness (in the case of several relevant authorities as well as the general public) of the threat that counterfeit medicines pose, if they exist at all.

Public health impact and pharmaco-vigilance

The types of adverse drug reaction (ADR) associated with the inadvertent use of counterfeit medicines can relate to one or more of a number of problems, depending on the type of counterfeiting practice employed. Counterfeit-medicine-associated ADRs may be due to, but not limited to, inappropriate API dose (absent, insufficient or excess dose) and quality problems (product contamination, excipient problems).

Under-reporting of possible counterfeit-medicine-related ADRs is likely to be significant when one takes into account the well-known problem of ADR under-reporting, even for authorised medicinal products. A weakness in the existing European pharmaco-vigilance system is that it is not explicitly geared to detection of 'drug ineffectiveness'. The direct impact of the inadvertent use of counterfeit medicines on public health in Europe by an unsuspecting public is thus difficult to determine based on known currently available data. While it is extremely unlikely that inadvertent consumption of counterfeit medicines in Europe is related to major mortality (unlike the situation that exists in some countries in Asia and Africa), it is certainly possible, if not probable, that counterfeit medicines make a not insignificant morbidity contribution (via, for example, ineffectiveness, inappropriate/inaccurate labelling and no possibility of batch recall).

Box 4 Types of medicinal product counterfeited

Product-market features

High volume (high level of prescribing)
High price (non-reimbursed, high price differential)
Known brand ('blockbusters')
Lifestyle (embarrassment/stigmatised) drugs
Unauthorised drugs
Drugs with off-label use indications
Drugs in short supply
Parenterals (in less developed/regulated countries)

Developed world

Branded drugs for erectile dysfunction (Viagra, Cialis) and weight loss (Reductil), cholesterol lowering agents (Lipitor), erythropoietins (Epo, Epogen, Neupogen, Procrit), anti-ageing (HGH), antibiotics (Augmentin) and antivirals (Tamiflu)

Developing world

Generic antibiotics, anti-malarials (e.g. Artusenate), vaccines and HIV drugs

Types of medicinal product counterfeited

Box 4 lists the types of medicinal product counterfeited, according to the responses received in the CoE survey, in terms of their product-market features and geographic placement.

No type of medicinal product appears to be exempt from being a counterfeiting target, although the types of medicinal product at higher risk of being counterfeited depend on the market characteristics of particular geographic regions. Although so-called 'lifestyle' (including 'embarrassment'/stigmatised) and essential drugs tend to be targets for counterfeiting in developed and developing countries respectively, this distinction in terms of product type by region is becoming increasingly blurred. It cannot be safely assumed that any particular class of medicinal product is immune from being counterfeited.

Pharmaceutical crime practices (medicines counterfeiting and diversion)

Box 5 presents a classification of pharmaceutical crime practices identified by survey respondents. These can be seen to be highly diverse, with no shortage of creativity shown by counterfeiters, particularly in the case of API counterfeiting. All these practices have been reported as occurring in Europe.

Factors behind the medicines counterfeiting phenomenon – system weaknesses and pharmaceutical crime

Europe is at risk from counterfeit medicines owing to a number of interrelated factors, as summarised in Box 6 on pages 14–15 and discussed below.

API manufacturing control and regulation

The evidence suggests that API regulatory control is an area of major weakness. For example, it is not beyond the realm of possibility that legitimate finished medicinal product (FP) manufacturers could unwittingly be marketing counterfeit

Box 5 Medicinal product counterfeiting and diversion practices

1 Finished medicinal products

1.1 Identical copy – identical formulation with packaging and labelling that are hard to differentiate from original

1.2 Pure counterfeit – altered/replaced ingredients with similar packaging (but either no/different/wrong dose, API or excipient)

1.3 Hybrid counterfeits:

Reuse of components/refilling – e.g. genuine containers (ampoules, bottles, vials, syringes)/packaging with substitute or no API

Illegal relabelling/repackaging – genuine formulated product falsely repackaged/relabelled as being from the original manufacturer and intended for the same or diverted to a different market from that originally intended by manufacturer (also includes use of fake pricing labels); includes products wrongly claiming to be an original product (e.g. use of well-known name or trademark)

1.4 Diversion and illegal trade of genuine medicinal products with genuine packaging and labelling (whether or not through the Internet)

1.5 Unpackaged medicinal products – e.g. wholesale/retail of medicinal products without the primary packaging

1.6 Placing a non-authorised medicinal product on the market

1.7 False documentation – e.g. granting a Certificate of Suitability (CoS or CEP)[1] by regulatory authorities without the given company being audited, false CEP, incorrect status on import documentation

1.8 False MAA – entire marketing applications sold and used; their contents do not have any relationship with the actual operations involved in the manufacture of the API or dosage form

1.9 Waste/expired product re-entering the market – includes repackaging and relabelling of expired products

2 Active pharmaceutical ingredients and excipients

2.1 API procurement from uncontrolled/non-GMP origin – done by some authorised FP manufacturers because uncontrolled API source is cheaper

2.2 Illegal API relabelling/repackaging – unauthorised API material may also be shipped in containers labelled with the name of a different API

2.3 'Ghost API manufacturing plant' – API (possibly not produced via the registered manufacturing process) not manufactured by the 'registered producer' is sold to FP MAH (who may be unaware of this fact, as API label mentions only the authorised manufacturer; a broker/trader may play a crucial role in this practice)

2.4 'Ghost API supplier' – MAH purchases API willingly and knowingly from a different manufacturer from that specified in the MA (in this case the manufacturing process will normally differ from that described and authorised in the MA)

2.5 'Paper curtain' – API manufacture performed through different process from that specified in the MA (a double documentation system may be used at the manufacturing site: one hidden set containing the true data and another set containing faked data that comply with authority requirements and regulations; such documentation systems may even be in place at a site where the API is not manufactured at all)

2.6 *'Authorised facades'* – manufacturer/trader with approved CEP and DMF supplies API material from a large number of unauthorised manufacturers (all labelling mentions only the authorised manufacturer. This set-up is believed to be widespread in terms of API material imported from China and possibly also India. In addition forged CoA and other forged documents will also be used in such situations)

2.7 *Illicit intermediate production* – unauthorised API materials from obscure sources are blended with the registered API material

medicines (either because the APIs utilised are fake or, if not fake, have a different specification to what was originally authorised).

In Europe, regulation of API manufacture and distribution is conducted at a much less intense level than for FPs. The types of control, where they exist, are highly variable and inconsistent between European states. Often there are no satisfactory regulatory controls of APIs (for example, manufacturing and broker/trader licensing and inspection, documentation validation, batch traceability and import/export/transit control) whatsoever. Thus it becomes all too easy for uncontrolled APIs (and excipients) to enter the legal manufacturing process.

Box 6 Factors facilitating the market entry of counterfeit medicines in Europe

- Lack of awareness and perception of the problem at authority/stakeholder and consumer levels
- Regulatory gaps (particularly regulation of APIs, packaging, labelling and distribution chain)
- Weak export/transit regulations (import regulations are generally strong except in the context of Internet/mail order pharmacy)
- Lack of coordination and inconsistency of approach between relevant authorities both nationally and internationally (medicines counterfeiting is a cross-sectoral problem; frequent absence of a SPOC, regulatory weakness in one member state impacts on all – 'weakest link' issue)
- Inefficient cooperation between stakeholders (within the supply chain and between the supply chain and authorities)
- Regulatory body lack of resources and lack of prioritisation (particularly to follow-up reports on suspected counterfeit medicines)
- Weak/uncoordinated enforcement and inappropriate penal sanctions (but some countries now addressing this issue, e.g. Germany)
- Disparity in legal availability between states of certain high-value innovative medicinal products (unlicensed medicines issue)

- Major price discrimination of medicinal products between European states (single European trade market but divergent health financing principles and systems)
- Rapid rise in Internet pharmacy trade (hardly regulated at all)
- Increasingly complex supply chain (with transactions involving many intermediaries)
- Recent historical appearance on the market of and demand for 'lifestyle' and 'embarrassment' drugs
- Increasing sophistication in clandestine manufacture

Trade and distribution

Pharmaceutical import, export and transit regulation and customs control

A number of important weaknesses exist.

In relation to import, export and transit controls on FPs, controls on APIs and bulk/intermediate products (BPs) are much less stringent and also inconsistent in Europe. As a result of the single EU market there is a limited requirement for trade controls between member states; thus APIs (and FPs) that have illicitly entered one state can then be easily disseminated throughout the EU.

The storage of pharmaceuticals in a bonded warehouse/free zone is inconsistently legislated for in European states.

Existing certification schemes in Europe are often inadequate, with large scope for documentation fraud (a 'reliance on paper' can be said to be important, but in comparison the

US FDA uses this and other methods to corroborate data – for example, use of E-data).

The actual factors and approach adopted by European states in medicinal product customs risk analysis and control are highly variable. Risk factors applying to medicinal products (for example, specific drug class or custom tariff code) are not universally employed by authorities. Very often customs will be heavily reliant upon information or intelligence provided by the right-holder. The types of control carried out by customs are often not specifically related to medicinal products, with the exception of narcotics and psychotropics, as a result of obligations under UN conventions (UN Conventions on Narcotic Drugs, 1961, Psychotropic Substances 1971, Illicit Traffic in Narcotic Drugs and Psychotropic Substances, 1988).

As a result of the single EU market, weaknesses in the trade control system of one member state can lead to a critical weak point in the entire EU pharmaceutical regulatory system. Thus, although some member states, with strong regulatory and control systems, may assume that they have no counterfeit medicine problem on their territory, this assumption may well be false.

Regulation of packaging, labelling, printing and parallel importation

Increasing supply-chain complexity (see below) is associated with ever more prevalent repackaging and relabelling practices, which are sometimes multiple for one product. Regulation of medicines (re)packaging, (re)labelling and printing is not performed consistently across European states. Of concern is the probable existence of unregulated or illegal packaging, labelling and printing facilities.

Legal provisions governing parallel importation (PI) in the EU tend to rely on existing provisions governing import licensing and marketing authorisation. As the regulation of FP PI is not determined at EU level, there is broad scope for member states to interpret their own procedures for governing PI.

The existence of a significant level of PI within the EU, in the absence of adequate controls on repackaging and relabelling, can inadvertently facilitate entry of counterfeit medicines from one member state into another; FP re- (exchangeable) packaging and labelling practices are highly prevalent across all European states.

Although known cases of counterfeit medicines have arisen in the European parallel trading system, the extent to which the practice of PI in itself is a facilitating factor for the dissemination of counterfeit medicines throughout Europe has not been sufficiently studied to draw any firm conclusions. What is clear, though, is that PI is reliant on a significant amount of repackaging, relabelling and printing, and contributes to the increasingily complex pharmaceutical distribution system in Europe.

Internet and mail-order pharmacy, unlicensed medicines and medicinal product advertising

Unquestionably, the Internet poses a significant risk in terms of the dissemination of counterfeit medicines, as there is little regulation of Internet medicines sales in Europe. The Internet, as well as mail order, offers an easy way to illegally distribute prescription-only and unlicensed medicines to consumers, and websites also offer for sale BPs. Internet pharmacy is possibly the leading type of 'spam' worldwide, with an emphasis on the retail of cheaper, lifestyle or unauthorised prescription medicines. As long as there is, first, an Internet and mail-order supply (without the need to obtain a prescription) and demand for these types of medicines and, second, a lack of public awareness of the risk of purchasing drugs through unregulated sources, this type of business will continue to thrive. Unregulated Internet and mail-order pharmacy of prescription drugs is a serious threat to public health and undermines the entire pharmaceutical regulatory framework. Under existing European legislation, health and pharmaceutical regulatory authorities are very often powerless to investigate and control this type of business.

Pharmaceutical/chemical brokers and traders

Although brokers and traders play an important role in the supply of APIs and BPs, there is little in the way of substantive evidence to suggest that they are a major contributory factor to the supply of counterfeit medicines. As facilitators of international commerce of medicines, brokers are, however, well placed to participate in the diversion of medicines, including counterfeits, as they lie outside the pharmaceutical regulatory system and remain invisible to authorities. Brokers are not directly subject to national legislation, they operate at an international level without being mentioned on bills and they are not a responsible party in the strict legislative sense. Brokers appear to be the only intermediaries in the pharmaceutical supply chain not subject to authorisation and regulatory control, which has to be a major point of concern.

The pharmaceutical distribution chain

Evidence exists that counterfeit medicines appear in the legal distribution chain at all stages. The reasons as to how they get there are probably several, and include insufficient distribution controls, multiple ownership and levels in the distribution chain, illegal trading by legal wholesalers and pharmacies, unregulated repackaging, sub-standard control practices by participants, documentation weaknesses and forgery, poor traceability requirements, and the relative ease of switching of legitimate to counterfeit API. In some countries, wholesalers and pharmacists report to different regulatory bodies, which makes regulation of the legal distribution chain more problematical.

Even in European states that have strong pharmaceutical regulation there is cause for concern in the legal distribution chain. A recent study by the Dutch Health Care Inspectorate (IGZ, 2005) revealed several major shortcomings in the application of Good Distribution Practice (GDP) by legitimate parallel and 'full range' distributors, summarised in Box 7 overleaf.

Trade globalisation, the dropping of trade barriers/restrictions and PI have led to the legal pharmaceutical distribution chain in Europe becoming increasingly complex and involving many intermediaries; particularly downstream, with the appearance of micro-distributors (i.e. short-line wholesalers, secondary wholesalers and wholesaling retailers, small import/export firms, etc.). Arguably, the value-added of pharmaceutical PI is dubious (Kanavos et al., 2004) and serves only to complicate the European distribution system and make regulatory control more difficult.

While pharmaceutical trade liberalisation may provide

Box 7 Findings from the 2004 Dutch Health Care Inspectorate study of distributors

The study revealed that GDP is not universally observed. In many cases, the distributor does not adequately check the trading authorisation of its customers. Moreover, almost all distributors lack a formal system to identify and intercept counterfeit medicines.

In several cases, actual infringements of current legislation were observed. For example, some distributors had purchased pharmaceuticals from persons without the necessary authorisation to sell them. Similarly, a number of wholesalers were found to have supplied pharmaceutical products to persons who were not authorised to trade in them.

A further finding is that too few safeguards exist to ensure the proper destruction of medicines. In most cases, it was not possible to demonstrate that products returned for destruction had actually been processed in the incinerators as required.

consumer benefits, including greater choice and cheaper prices, it presents problems for the health regulatory authorities. First, the jurisdiction of the latter is confined within state borders, and second, the same authorities have understandable difficulties in applying the prescribed principles of Good Trade and Distribution Practice (GTDP) to distributors below the level of the primary distributor. Criminal organisations and dishonest traders can easily take advantage of this situation.

The 'unregulated'/illegal distribution chain feeds off the legal distribution system via the practice of diversion; it undoubtedly plays a major role in the distribution of counterfeit medicines and is made up of a diverse range of players. These include secondary wholesalers and wholesaling pharmacies and entities such as fitness and bodybuilding clubs, shops specialising in undercover goods of all types, illegal wholesalers and retailers (following Internet bulk purchasing), sex clubs/shops, and food supplement and cosmetic stores.

Medicinal product security and traceability (pedigree tracking) systems

Current security and traceability systems are generally regarded as being weak in their capacity to counteract the increasing sophistication in original packaging (and dosage form) forgery and to cope with the increasingly complex distribution system. What is particularly worrying is that, compared with FPs, security and traceability systems for APIs and BPs are arguably practically non-existent. Concerning product security, several companies are now examining the possibility of introducing systems that consist of one or more overt, covert or forensic features, including trace substances, more unique closure systems and infrared spectrographic methods. Concerning traceability, proposals include the introduction of authentication technology for rapid identification at the pharmacy level, Internet-based track and trace, mandatory paper or electronic pedigree, bar coding and radio frequency identification tagging (RFID).

Currently absent, though, in Europe are unified and harmonised regulatory guidelines that can assist manufacturers in defining a common minimal security and traceability standard and which can assist European regulatory authorities in their task.

Legislative, penal and enforcement provisions

No single satisfactory coherent national legal provision against medicines counterfeiting exists in Europe. Potentially applicable legislative provisions are horizontal and non-specific to counterfeit medicines and tend to be incorporated into one or more different sector-specific laws and regulations (i.e. laws governing medicinal products, penal or criminal provisions, customs and trade or intellectual property). These potentially applicable legal provisions exhibit a large degree of diversity between European states and often weak inter-sectoral legislative coordination. Many stakeholders would like to see counterfeit-medicine-specific legislation enacted.

A corollary of the inconsistent situation described above is that this leads to the problems of authority sectoral lack of coordination and incoherence both at the state and the European level, and thus difficulties for effectively tackling counterfeit medicines.

In the overwhelming majority of European states no clear definitions of 'counterfeit medicine' and 'pharmaceutical crime' exist. Frequently such definitions can only be implied indirectly. The absence of commonly agreed and utilised definitions and coherent legal provisions against medicines counterfeiting in Europe leads to inconsistencies and non-standardisation of case reporting by both authorities and stakeholders, and thus the difficulty of obtaining an accurate overall picture of the counterfeit medicine situation. It also reinforces the perception that medicines counterfeiting is no different from other types of product counterfeiting (a fallacy in view of the public health consequences).

In Europe, criminal sanctions are in place for product counterfeiting in general as a result of applicable IPR law, but they are far from being harmonised between states. Owing to the territorial limitation of national IPR laws, counterfeiters can exploit the discrepancies between states in order to escape or minimise the risk of criminal sanctions. Frequently a confounding problem is the prosecution of counterfeiters outside the territory where the products are placed.

A further weakness of the IPR protection system in Europe is that generic drugs are particularly badly protected by legislation in its present form. It has been proposed that there should be some form of expired patent rights relay applied to generic drugs in order to deter counterfeiting of the latter.

With possibly a few exceptions, no specific sanctions are applied against medicines counterfeiting, the latter generally regarded as being purely an economic crime as opposed to both an economic and a health crime. Consequently, existing sanctions for medicines counterfeiting are too feeble to deter their manufacture and distribution by dishonest traders and criminal organisations. Sanctions are far too light given the threat to human well-being and health system security that counterfeit medicines pose. Some European states, however (for example, Germany; Wesch, 2004), are now beginning to recognise the need to differentiate medicines counterfeiting and health crime from other forms of counterfeiting and crime and are revising their legislation accordingly.

In recognition of the fact that currently applicable IPR sanctions are weak, in 2005 the EC proposed a directive that

Box 8 Justification for the proposed EC Directive 'On criminal measures aimed at ensuring the enforcement of intellectual property rights'

'The disparities between the national systems of penalties, apart from hampering the proper functioning of the internal market, make it difficult to combat counterfeiting and piracy effectively. In addition to the economic and social consequences, counterfeiting and piracy also pose problems for consumer protection, particularly when health and safety are at stake. Increasing use of the Internet enables pirated products to be distributed instantly around the globe. Finally, this phenomenon appears to be increasingly linked to organised crime. Combating this phenomenon is therefore of vital importance for the Community.' (EC, 2005)

lays down the criminal measures necessary to ensure IPR enforcement (EC, 2005; Box 8 above describes the justification for this proposed directive).[2]

Once the required sanctions are put in place, it is then necessary to enforce them. In Europe, the quality of enforcement of sanctions against medicines counterfeiting presents a mixed picture. For a number of reasons inspection and enforcement are often weak, for example through a lack of power and coordination. Some states may have provided for sanctions which, however, would be difficult or take too long to implement in their courts.

Administrative weaknesses

To effectively combat medicines counterfeiting in Europe requires an effective administrative system geared to tackling the problem. Unfortunately in Europe this is absent; there is a large degree of administrative lack of coordination and structural complexity at all levels, which equates with a 'system failure' and which is a situation freely admitted by the majority of relevant authorities and legitimate manufacturers and distributors.

Some major coordination gaps exist between authorities in the different relevant sectors at a national level and between similar authorities in different countries. If the counterfeit medicine problem is recognised for the large problem both in public health and in economic terms that it is, then serious efforts need to be made to increase national inter-sectoral cooperation, preferably on a formalised basis.

Legal provisions for reporting of counterfeit medicines are mostly absent in Europe (as are corresponding provisions for confidentiality of reporting), and where they do exist the types of provision are highly variable. Thus, unsurprisingly, there are large data incongruencies between counterfeit medicine cases known to various sectoral national authorities, manufacturers and wholesalers.

The several reasons why European administrations perform poorly in dealing with counterfeit medicines include the following: the issue has not been placed on national agendas; there is often low awareness among authorities of the existence of a counterfeit medicine problem in Europe (there may also be an element of complacency and regulatory denial); detection and inspection systems are often inadequate; analytical testing procedures are unclear; reporting systems tend to be informal and often with no clear single point of contact nationally or at a European level; there is an absence of centralised and fully utilised counterfeit medicine databases linked to regulatory enforcement;[3] there is unclear sectoral authority (i.e. police, health or trade) jurisdiction over counterfeit medicines; different countries have different administrative organisational set-ups; data confidentiality and disclosure procedures provide impediments to effective communication; often states desire to maintain control over national jurisdiction; the European pharmaceutical regulatory system is in transition;[4] and finally the fact that the EU is going through a major stage of growth and administrative construction owing largely to its recent round of expansion.

In the absence of formal administrative systems and procedures, medicines counterfeiting is currently dealt with via ad hoc national arrangements and a plethora of ill-coordinated organisations. Uncoordinated and informal approaches are not effective. What is clear is that the absence of national-level coordinating bodies (and arguably also of a European-level coordinating body) greatly hinders the possibility of taking effective action against medicines counterfeiting.

Pharmaceutical crime

In Europe, authorities are struggling to cope with the growing threats posed by the increasing sophistication of organised crime (Newton-Dunn, 2004) and counterfeiting in general (CEIPI, 2004). Strong evidence exists that medicines counterfeiting is linked with organised crime. Counterfeiting of medicines is a lucrative business owing to the high demand for medicines and low production costs.

In many ways pharmaceutical crime can be viewed as a natural extension (or 'business diversification') of illicit narcotic and psychotropic drug manufacturing and distribution. Experience with illicit narcotic and psychotropic production lends itself to increasing sophistication in clandestine manufacture of medicinal products.

With respect to illicit API production, a strong indicator of API counterfeiting is the existence of very small companies (with around fifty employees) that claim to manufacture hundreds of different APIs and sell them under their own label as if being manufactured by that company.

Where do counterfeit medicines placed on the European market originate from? Organised criminal gangs from the former Soviet Union and Balkans are known to be involved in the pharmaceutical crime business and manufacturing sites are either within these regions or outside Europe, sited in countries such as China and India that have weak pharmaceutical regulatory and enforcement structures.

As Box 5 shows (see p. 11), pharmaceutical crime is a creative business. Pharmaceutical criminals take maximum advantage of the deficiencies and loopholes in the international pharmaceutical trading, regulatory, legislative and administrative systems. Pharmaceutical crime is assisted by increasing sophistication in clandestine manufacture and a lack of knowledge and understanding by authorities of the 'pharmaceutical crime business model'.

As stated in the essay 'Europe needs an FBI', 'if details of organised crime operations in Europe are vague it is because they are so by definition – organised gangs keep themselves hidden, hence information about them is scarce. Many base themselves outside of the European Union. Organised crime crosses frontiers in Europe effortlessly, but police forces and legal jurisdictions are national' (Newton-Dunn, 2004). This report goes on to say that urgent improvements to law enforcement across Europe are required (particularly inter-state coordination) and that ideally international crime in Europe should be fought by a European-level law enforcement agency. There has been a great deal of speculation as to the possibility of Europol becoming a European version of the FBI. Despite the considerable advantages that such a set-up would bring, however, there are a number of obstacles that would need to be overcome in order for such a transformation to take place.[5]

Irrespective of the merits or otherwise of establishing a European-level law enforcement agency, certainly it is now recognised that law enforcement at the state level needs strengthening in order to cope with the increasing sophistication of organised crime in Europe. For example, the UK has very recently gone ahead with the establishment of its Serious Organised Crime Agency (see Box 9).

Proposed solutions for Europe

Just prior to and in the intervening year since completion and final publication of the CoE report, a number of further reports on the counterfeit medicine problem have surfaced (e.g. Satchwell, 2004; O'Mathuna and McAuley, 2005), which reflect the growing and necessary attention that this subject is now receiving. The CoE report, *inter alia*, has provided significant evidence that a counterfeit medicine problem exists in Europe; thus from a political perspective the problem now deserves

Box 9 The UK Serious Organised Crime Agency (SOCA)

Tony Blair says a new force will tackle the 'brutal and sophisticated' criminal gangs of the 21st century. The Serious Organised Crime Agency, dubbed Britain's FBI, will bring together more than 4,000 police, customs and immigration experts. Soca 'law enforcement officers', with new multiple powers, will target international drug and people traffickers and fraudsters. They would make life 'hell' for 'Mr Bigs', Mr Blair said at Soca's launch. 'The level of sophistication, the level, frankly, of brutality with which many of these gangs operate today means that we have to do it differently,' Mr Blair said at the Downing Street launch.

Soca amalgamates the National Crime Squad, the National Criminal Intelligence Service (NCIS), and investigators from Customs and the Home Office's Immigration Service. A major part of its role is to 'reduce harm' to members of the public which will be measured by indicators such as falls in robberies or the number of addicts in treatment. Initially, it also aims to build up more comprehensive intelligence on organised crime networks operating in the UK.

Mr Blair said the agency would exploit four important new powers:

- Queen's evidence: Prosecutors will be able to offer statutory deals – immunity or reduced sentences – where, previously, deals were only informal
- Financial reporting orders: Courts can make orders, of up to 20 years, forcing criminals to provide bank statements to ensure they have no crime-related earnings

- Disclosure notices: Courts can force suspects to answer questions or provide documents or face imprisonment or fines. Limits the right to silence
- Law enforcement officers: Soca officers will have the multiple powers of police, immigration (BBC News, 2006)

serious consideration. On a positive note, at the European political level this problem is now receiving serious consideration; first by the CoE itself (2004) and now by the EC (2006). Whether medicines counterfeiting is a passing phenomenon of today or here to stay largely depends on the political will and actions to be taken by those in a position to do so.

At the international level, the WHO continues to further its important leadership role in addressing the global counterfeit medicine problem. Recently, at the WHO Rome International Conference 'Combating counterfeit drugs: building effective international collaboration' (WHO, 2006b), the participants formulated a declaration that recognises that combating counterfeit medicines requires (i) the coordinated effort of all the different public and private stakeholders that are affected and are competent to address the different aspects of the problem, and (ii) effective coordination and cooperation at the international level in order for regional and national strategies to be more effective.

To achieve these objectives it was resolved that the WHO should lead the establishment of an International Medical Products Anti-counterfeiting Taskforce (IMPACT) of governmental, non-governmental and international institutions on the basis of existing institutions. In the long term it was proposed that further mechanisms should be explored (including the possibility of an international convention) for strengthening international action against counterfeit medicines.

There are no simple solutions to what is a problem with complex causality. An effective solution for Europe requires a number of interrelated and coordinated measures, as proposed in Box 10 on pages 32–3.

In Europe, given that counterfeit medicines and pharmaceutical crime are a cross-border problem and that large-scale lack of coordination is probably the most fundamental problem hindering effective counteraction, there is strong justification for the adoption of a Europe-level binding instrument that provides the legislative framework to effectively tackle medicines counterfeiting. Whether or not there should be a specific piece of counterfeit medicines/pharmaceutical crime legislation (or sub-law) very much depends on the analysis of a detailed codification of potentially applicable legislation in the European states,[6] which should identify areas of legislative gaps and lack of coordination. It is worth stating that some countries (not in Europe) have implemented counterfeit-medicine-specific legislation (e.g. Republic of the Philippines, 2003). An advantage of such an approach is that it rightly serves to differentiate medicines counterfeiting and health crime from other forms of counterfeiting that do not result in the same degree of risk to health.

A good model for whatever solution is eventually developed for Europe is provided by the UN International Narcotic Control Board (INCB) and its framework conventions that deal with the

Box 10 Key measures to combat medicines counterfeiting

1. European-lèvel binding instrument (highest form of legal cooperation possible, e.g. convention, directive)
2. European-level coordinating body (with clear definition of Europe- and state-level institutional roles and responsibilities), responsible for:
   - European state and national authority cross-sectoral coordination (SPOC)
   - Establishment and definition of communication networks, best practices, codes, protocols, relevant databases, reporting systems and information-sharing and disclosure procedures
   - Communication strategy (awareness- and knowledge-raising; improved information for general public, health professionals, supply chain participants and authorities)
3. Anti-CM/PC legislative framework/implementing tool (possibly specific to CM/PC):
   - Codification of possibly applicable European state legislation
   - Standardisation of important definitions (CM and PC) and rules of interpretation
   - Strengthening and implementation of regulations applicable to pharmaceutical/chemical brokers and traders (i.e. GDP and GTDP), Internet and mail-order pharmacy (FDA, 2004),[7] unlicensed medicines usage, (re)packaging, (re)labelling and printing, APIs[8] and excipients

- Risk management plan:
  - Active searching, inspection and analytical testing procedures
  - Security and traceability (pedigree tracking) systems
  - Rapid Alert System (RAS)
  - Pharmaco-vigilance (more explicit inclusion of CM under existing systems, targeting products with high risk of counterfeiting and health risk)
  - Customs control and risk analysis procedures specific to medicinal products
- IPR measures addressing CM (including extension to generics)
- Sanctions and penalties sufficient to deter medicine counterfeiters
- Customs and health authority information-sharing concerning suspected CM

4 Detailed characterisation of the CM criminal business model (manufacturing, distribution and retail)

5 Enforcement improvements (adoption of best European practices, e.g. pharmaceutical/health crime unit), strengthening of national law enforcement and possible establishment of European law enforcement agency

6 Training (health authorities, customs, law enforcement personnel, etc.) and public education

illicit drug trade (Single Convention on Narcotic Drugs, 1961). The INCB manages to effectively coordinate health, customs and law enforcement authorities at an international level, underpinned by the relevant international conventions.

Conclusions

A suitable way of summarising the counterfeit medicine situation in Europe and its potential solution is to place the factors behind this phenomenon under the headings of *invisibility, biohazard* and *system failure,* and then to present a European prescription.

Invisibility

There is an invisibility problem associated with medicines counterfeiting. How big the iceberg is in Europe no one can confidently say with any degree of accuracy. By the very nature of medicines, their counterfeits are harder to detect than counterfeits of other product types. By their own nature, the organised criminals that manufacturer and distribute counterfeit medicines are also hard to detect. A lack of awareness among several stakeholders, including the general public, of the prevalence of counterfeit medicines in Europe contributes towards this situation, one not helped by the relatively weak detection systems that exist in Europe. As the evidence begins to accumulate, it is now becoming more difficult for policy-makers and authorities in Europe to deny that medicines counterfeiting is a problem demanding attention. As discussed below, the invisibility factor leads to difficulty in determining the true 'biohazard' impact of counterfeit medicines and contributes to the failure of systems in Europe to adequately address the problem.

Biohazard

In addition to the economic damage caused by counterfeiting, there is no question that counterfeit medicines put human health at risk and undermine the credibility of health systems. Although, first, pharmaceutical criminals do not in all likelihood set out with the intention of damaging public health and, second, it is unlikely that there is large-scale resultant mortality from consumption of counterfeit medicines in Europe, the fact that counterfeit medicines, by their very nature, are outside the regulatory system leaves major cause for concern. At the very least there is likely to be a not insignificant degree of morbidity arising from their consumption (via drug ineffectiveness and inappropriate labelling and patient information leading to misusage). The fact that pharmaco-vigilance systems suffer from a relative failure to detect drug ineffectiveness means that the actual extent of counterfeit-medicine-related morbidity is hard to determine. What is certain, though, is that one death from medicines counterfeiting in Europe is one death too many, and that policy-makers and authorities should do everything in their power to prevent this possibility. We should avoid complacency and be proactive in order to avoid the situation where necessary pharmaceutical regulatory development has to be prompted by a 'pharmageddon' scenario, as has sometimes historically been the case (FDA, 2001).

System failure

Medicines counterfeiting is a phenomenon of our time with

complex causality. Pharmaceutical market globalisation in the wake of trade liberalisation is a positive economic trend; without the necessary regulatory and enforcement infrastructure to support it, however, the situation is readily exploited by increasingly sophisticated organised criminals. The evidence and stakeholder commentary presented in the CoE report demonstrate that there are major weaknesses in relevant European regulation, legislation, enforcement and administration. In the EU, the complex and developing administrative structure and absorption pressure from new and potential member states are contributing factors. The extent to which parallel trade is also a contributing factor requires further study.

The European prescription

There is no simple solution to a complex problem, and it will take time to get the necessary prescription in place. The prescription ingredients consist of (i) political action and awareness-raising, (ii) regulatory, legislative and enforcement improvements, and (iii) an appropriate risk management system. These ingredients then require mixing together effectively via the establishment of both national and European-level coordinating bodies. Medicines counterfeiting is becoming an increasingly sophisticated activity which requires an equally sophisticated remedy. It is now time for politicians and authorities to get real with the threat posed by counterfeit medicines and pharmaceutical crime.

2

Facing the reality of medicines counterfeiting

What could and should European stakeholders in safe medicines supply be doing?

David Taylor

Introduction

The world pharmaceutical market is today worth in the order of $500 billion annually. About 80% of this expenditure – which is equivalent to a little under 1% of global GDP – takes place in the developed world, where 20% of the world's population lives. It is in rich countries that the opportunity for profiting from selling counterfeit medicines is potentially at its greatest. Yet presently it is in poorer countries such as India, China and those of sub-Saharan Africa that medicines counterfeiting is most prevalent, and where lives are most frequently being lost as a result. For example, children and adults are dying as a result of the supply of ineffective treatments for conditions such as malaria (Haines, 2006).

Western Europe, by contrast, has to date had a relatively strong record in defending the integrity of its pharmaceutical manufacturing and supply processes. Despite the size of its market (some 30% of all medicines by value are consumed in the EU today), the region's wealth and high level of social solidarity – and hence its capacity to invest in extensive regulatory systems and robustly professional pharmacy and medical care networks – have protected the public from the serious health hazards that counterfeit medicines use threatens. By contrast, the poverty of many communities in Africa and Asia can serve to promote corruption in health and other sectors (Transparency International, 2006) and to impair policing efforts. Such phenomena undermine economic growth, creating a vicious cycle of harm.

The complexity of the European medicines market, which has been characterised by both linguistic and administrative diversity, might also – perhaps paradoxically – have served to defend public health interests. Counterfeiters may have found it easier to produce and distribute fake products in larger, in some ways more unified, healthcare markets such as that of the United States, where a relatively large number of medicines-counterfeiting cases have been found (Satchwell, 2004). Additionally, the fact that US medicine consumers have relatively often to fund their pharmaceutical treatment out of their own pockets may have made them more likely than their western European counterparts to risk obtaining supplies via the Internet, or other vulnerable routes.

As contributors to a WHO conference on counterfeiting held in February 2006 in Rome emphasised, however, Europe cannot afford to be complacent. For example, Dr Nils Behrnt, a senior European Commission official, informed participants in this event that for the period 2000–05 alone he was aware of 27 separate counterfeit medicine supply events in the legitimate European supply chain (Behrnt, 2006). He also testified to knowledge of 170 cases in the illegitimate/non-legal supply chain in the same period. The latter may be exemplified by instances of people obtaining fake prescription medicines for conditions such as depression or erectile dysfunction via Internet-based suppliers.

Many EU agencies may not – at least until external pressures began to build in the last few years – have had reason assertively to prioritise the identification of counterfeiting cases. Hence such data can be seen as indicative of a potentially large future problem. Figures from sources such as the Council of Europe (Harper, 2006) also support this conclusion.

Against this background this chapter briefly explores the nature of the medicines-counterfeiting threat now facing the European Union. It examines a range of social and economic policy issues relating to it, and the (sometimes conflicting) interests of European stakeholders in pharmaceutical innovation, production, supply and use. The scale and changing characteristics of the pharmaceutical market in Europe are initially outlined. This is followed by a short analysis of stakeholder interests, and a discussion of key medicine-related policy and policy research issues that Europe and its partners need to address in the early 21st century. The conclusion seeks to summarise an answer to the question '*What could and should European stakeholders in safe medicines supply be doing about medicines counterfeiting?*'

But before this a final set of introductory points is noted. They relate to the fact that public debate on health and other policy matters can fail to promote progress because of the dangers of oversimplification on the one hand and the temptations of exaggeration or denial on the other. In the context of pharmaceutical counterfeiting, for example, it would be relatively easy to communicate alarmist messages to the effect that large numbers of European Union citizens are at imminent risk of being harmed owing to the use of fake, sub-standard or even positively toxic medicinal drugs. Yet this – to date, at least – is not the case. A more difficult political message to communicate would be that although dangers to public health per se from medicine counterfeiting are currently limited, it would be prudent to take a precautionary approach and initiate action now to control a potentially important future problem.

An even more difficult message to communicate to policy-making and other audiences would be that the counterfeit drugs issue – although a genuinely serious cause for concern – might in some instances be best regarded as an indicator of the existence of more important, long-term threats to European public interests. These are in part linked to the desirability or otherwise of policies that encourage the use of generic medicines (which, although low-cost, may from a patient perspective be unrecognisable) and the parallel trading of patented medicines within Europe. This last practice – which in US terminology is often referred to as drug reimportation – entails the repackaging and reselling of medicines bought at a low (governmentally controlled) price in one EU member state and then resupplied at a higher (also officially permitted) price elsewhere in the Union. This process can involve products passing through twenty or thirty transactions between their source and their eventual supply to a patient.

Wider questions linked to medicines-counterfeiting hazards and the pursuit of 'cheap drug deals' by pharmacists and traders relate to how in a changing global economy Europe hopes to maintain the living standards of its people, and fulfil their desire not only for affordable healthcare today but also for better, more effective future treatments. The most important topics to be addressed in this context are about how Europe can continue to fund and undertake medicine and other forms of biomedical research in an effective and collectively beneficial manner.

Europe's pharmaceutical heritage, and current challenges to its maintenance

American-owned pharmaceutical companies are today responsible on an aggregated annual basis for over 50% of all new medicinal-entity-based drugs introduced globally. In absolute terms, and proportionately to the size of its economy, the USA spends more both publicly and privately on pharmaceutical and other forms of biomedical research than does the EU or any of its individual member states.

Yet Europe as a region still employs more people in its pharmaceutical industry than does the USA. The European pharmaceutical sector offers some 600,000 jobs, and the EU enjoys a positive balance of trade in medicines with the rest of the world of nearly €40 billion (EFPIA, 2006). Such statistics indicate that several million European households presently derive their income, directly or indirectly, from pharmaceutical research and manufacturing.

Within the boundaries of Europe, Ireland is arguably the most successful medicines producer. It has a net balance of internal EU pharmaceutical trade of around €14 billion. This compares with an equivalent figure of around €6 billon in France, €4 billion in the UK and a small net deficit in Germany. (Irish commentators have also acknowledged the existence of a local as well as a global medicines-counterfeiting threat; O'Mathuna and McAuley, 2005).

The European pharmaceutical sector is presently facing a number of challenges. They range from the emergence of low-cost manufacturing competition in Eastern countries such as China and India to the rising cost and increasing difficulty of conducting clinical and other research in the EU. Research-based pharmaceutical companies are investing more in innovation than at any previous time. In terms of generating new treatment concepts they also appear to be as – or more – creative than ever before. But the rate at which new ideas and knowledge are being translated into economically successful new products is at a nadir.

This reality – which is partly a function of regulatory interventions – has helped to drive mergers within the pharmaceutical industry. So too in Europe have supply-side controls on medicine prices, coupled with demand-side restrictions on prescribing choices and budgets. Encouraging the parallel importing of medicines is arguably a facet of the latter.

The overall economic impacts of such interventions are uncertain. This is to a degree because short-term savings could translate into long-term costs for the overall European economy. The available evidence on parallel importing suggests that to date, even though something like 140 million medicine packs are traded via this route annually, the total savings generated for EU healthcare funders have been limited (Kanavos et al., 2005). They appear to be in the order of €1–2 billion in a European pharmaceutical market worth well over €100 billion, and against an overall level of healthcare investment of over €1,000 billion per annum.

The economic impact on research-based pharmaceutical companies operating in settings such as the UK, however, where in value terms one medicine in every five used is a parallel import, should not be underestimated. For every euro saved by healthcare providers such as the NHS through the use of pharmaceutical parallel imports, research-based companies may lose around three. This is because of costs incurred and profits taken in the chains of commercial and professional traders involved.

It would be incorrect to allege that licensed parallel import medicine traders are directly responsible for facilitating the introduction of counterfeit medicines into the EU, or that generic medicines licensed in Europe are biomedically inferior to their branded counterparts. But equally it would be wrong to deny that the growth of complex patterns of trading in medicines in Europe has extended medicine supply chains in ways that increase opportunities for criminals to introduce fake products. This point is illustrated in Figure 1. It describes the convoluted trading sequences involved in the supply of a fake anti-obesity product in the UK eventually found to have been distributed nationwide (Anderson, 2006). Similarly, it would be disingenuous to suggest that the dispensing of ever-changing generic medicine presentations does not weaken their users' ability to identify errors and abnormalities.

A final point to stress in this context is that the European Union has recently expanded. It is continuing to change culturally as well as economically. As its borders extend eastwards to include populations that are relatively poor and which are

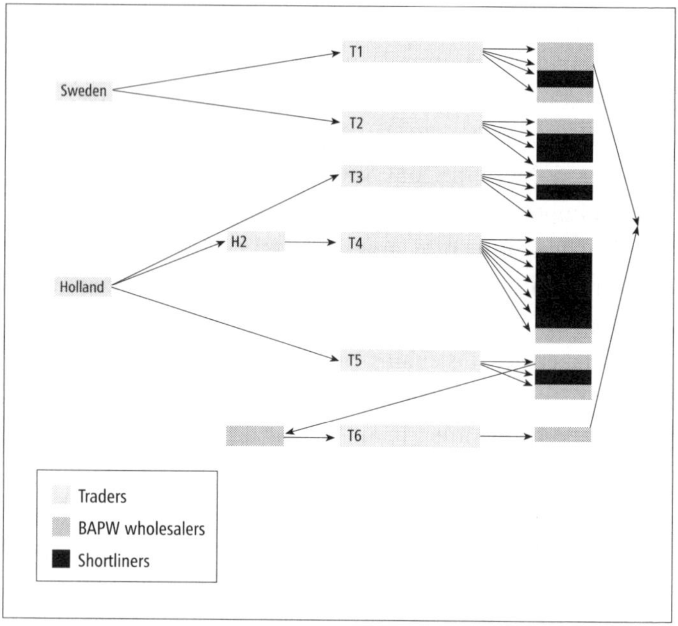

Figure 1 An illustrative counterfeit product flow through the European/UK medicines supply chain

served by healthcare systems less comprehensive than those found in the pre-2004 Union, the risk of fake treatments entering legitimate and illegitimate medicine supply chains is likely to grow. Russia is reportedly a major producer of counterfeit pharmaceuticals.

If the integrity of the EU's pharmaceutical supply chain is seriously impaired, it will only be after a period of time that this will become fully apparent in terms of potentially avoidable deaths. One vital policy question this prospect raises relates to whether or not European politicians and regulators have taken needless risks in facilitating perceived (if in reality only minor) cash savings for healthcare funders, while at the same time driving up the costs of pharmaceutical innovation through an excess of caution in other contexts.

Stakeholder interests

All legitimate stakeholders in the European medicines market have an interest in maintaining, and where possible improving, the safety of medicines supply and use, and so overall public health. Even criminals involved in trading in fake drugs are unlikely to wish deliberately to cause harm, albeit that the nature of their activities will inevitably increase risks. Hazard levels will be raised even when counterfeits are intended to contain the correct active ingredients, not least because they cannot be recalled if a manufacturing mistake is discovered.

The most important pharmaceutical stakeholder group is the medicine-using public. Taxpayers and patients have complex and sometimes conflicting interests in this field. In essence, resolving consequent tensions involves making trade-offs between maximising current welfare levels and investing in future well-being. The latter may take the form of employment for the young, or increased survival and freedom from disability for the elderly.

Defending the public's immediate and longer-term interests must also involve taking policy decisions about protecting populations from counterfeit medicines on the one hand, and permitting increasing freedom of (self- as well as professionally managed) treatment access and choice on the other. The contrasting (liberal) US and (conservative) EU approaches to allowing private companies to provide information about prescription medicines directly to the public illustrate the dilemmas to be faced in this field, as does the issue of controlling Internet trading.

Within European civil society the main institutional public and private stakeholders in safe medicines supply include:

- **the European Commission and associated supranational agencies.** A major goal for many supporters of 'the European project' is to extend the single market, and eliminate national-level differences that inhibit trading and/or fragment governance across the Union. Hence the Commission has (notwithstanding recent initiatives following the publication of the 'G10' report – see www.pharmacos.eudra.org/g10/docs/G10-Medicines.pdf) tended to promote parallel importing of medicines in the name of free trade, regardless of whether or not it may complicate pharmaceutical supply lines. Yet in reality opportunities for parallel trading in European medicines are a function of disparate member-state-level price-fixing interventions. Similarly, the perceived interests of individuals and groups concerned primarily with strengthening the European single market may not in practice include fostering research excellence, if this involves preserving national-level arrangements seen as inhibiting 'ever closer union';
- **EU member state governments, and national-level regulatory and allied health sector management agencies such as medicine licensing and safety monitoring organisations.** Politicians in member states with a weak pharmaceutical research base and low

numbers of pharmaceutical sector jobs may require lower prices for new pharmaceuticals than those with greater (electoral) interests in this area. At the same time local regulatory agencies may well be concerned with their survival, not least because medicines licensing in Europe has increasingly become a Union function. Managing the threat from fake medicines could from this perspective be seen as an important area for extended future activity at member state level, even if past practices have not always been as rigorous as they might have been. (See, for instance, Carlton, 2006.) With regard to the possible risks of parallel importing, member-state-level officials are likely to believe that politicians see this activity as saving public money. Hence they may conclude that it is in their best interests to defend pharmaceutical parallel importing, regardless of other considerations;

- **pharmaceutical companies and representative organisations funded by both research-based and generic medicine producers/suppliers.** Research-based and generic medicine manufacturers share common interests in supplying high-quality and effective medicines, and retaining the confidence of their customers at all points in the medicines value and supply chain outlined in Figure 2. All legitimate pharmaceutical producers are therefore concerned to prevent counterfeiting, albeit that for criminals operating in Europe the greatest profits are to be made from copying branded and/or patent-protected products (sales of which fund research and promotion) rather than lower-cost generic medicines. Research-based pharmaceutical companies also have interests in drawing attention to the risks and (for them in particular) the financial damage associated with pharmaceutical parallel importing/reimportation, both in Europe and (potentially) the USA. Some companies, however, may wish not to publicise counterfeiting incidents involving their products for fear of undermining their reputation. A minority may even seek to avoid publicity being given to any case of medicines counterfeiting;

- **pharmaceutical wholesalers and parallel traders.** All legitimate suppliers of medicines also have powerful reasons to guard against counterfeiting. They have a commercial interest in seeking to ensure that fake products are excluded from every possible entry point into the European pharmaceutical supply chain. Pharmaceutical wholesaling is an increasingly concentrated industry in Europe, which operates at a highly sophisticated level (Taylor et al., 2004). Virtually all large European pharmaceutical wholesalers now supply parallel imports. Many small – sometimes little more than single-person – organisations also act, however, as traders in PI medicines throughout the expanded European Union. Over 5,000 European pharmaceutical parallel trading licences have now been issued. In some individual cases very small traders may represent weak points in the supply chain;
- **pharmacies and pharmacists.** Pharmacists have a professional duty to protect public interests in the safe supply and use of medicines. In EU countries such as the UK large pharmacy chains are vertically linked with wholesaling organisations, while throughout the Union a number of much smaller pharmacies are also licensed PI

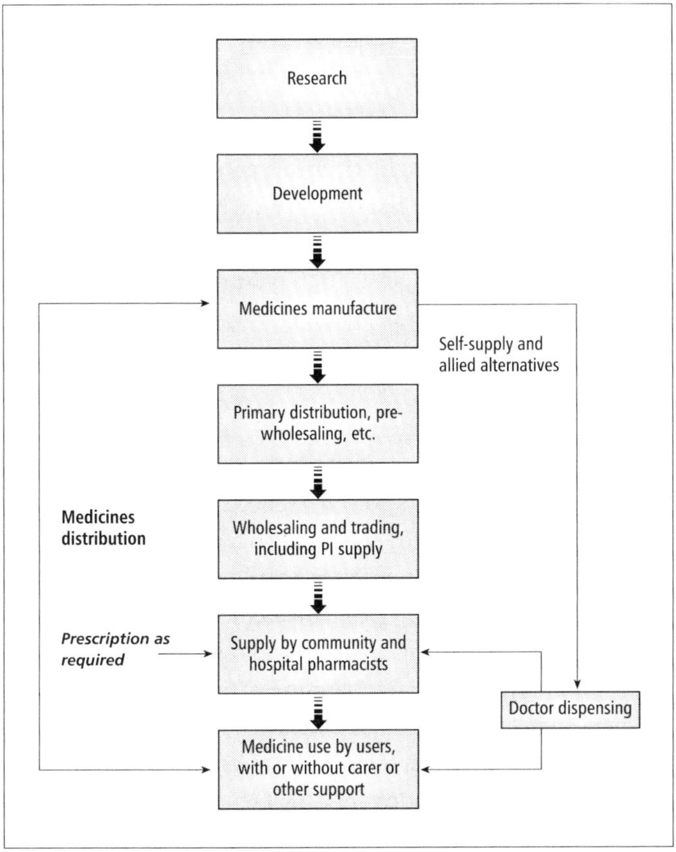

Figure 2 **The pharmaceutical value and supply chain in Europe**

traders. Large concerns and smaller pharmacies purchasing only from reputable wholesalers can normally guarantee that their customers will not be exposed to fake medicines. But where more vulnerable pharmacies are under financial pressure to purchase pharmaceutical products as cheaply as possible (as can be the case even in western Europe, in countries like Holland and the UK) the risk of counterfeits reaching the public may be exacerbated;

- **media and related organisations, such as political parties and academic institutions contributing to public debate.** Actors in this last category are not concerned directly with medicines supply. Rather, they trade in stories, concepts and policies relevant to pharmaceutical products and the sector as a whole, in order to gain money, status and power.

It would be beyond the scope of this brief paper to explore these last stakeholders' interests in further depth. One final point is worth stressing, however. It reflects warnings previously made about the difficulties associated with communicating complex arguments as opposed to simplified half-truths.

In relation to the European medicines supply chain and the factors that may have made it needlessly vulnerable to the risk of counterfeit medicines harming patients, it is commonly assumed that such developments have been necessary to save money. But this is in fact questionable. In the case of pharmaceutical parallel importing in the EU, for instance, a full cost–benefit analysis might well show that alternative strategies (perhaps involving freely set uniform prices, or prohibitions on the movement of differentially priced patented medicines across internal European borders) could have provided a more cost-effective way forward. To date, no comprehensive policy impact analysis – taking into account factors such as public interest in maintaining the viability of private sector mechanisms for funding biomedical research – has been completed.

A point to stress in this context is that it should not be uncritically assumed that only commercial companies seek profit. All stakeholders in any complex social function inevitably have sectional interests, and seek gain in one form or another. This includes public sector managers, regulators, journalists and politicians, whether or not they happen to own shares in private companies. Problems such as tackling medicines counterfeiting need to approached in the light of this understanding. So too do wider (but logically associated) challenges, such as ensuring that Europe invests adequately in biomedical research for its future health and wealth.

Policy issues and research questions

There are three main messages this chapter is seeking to communicate about medicines counterfeiting. They can be summarised as follows:

1. Drug counterfeiting is a major form of illicit enterprise. In regions such as South Asia and sub-Saharan Africa 'guesstimates' of the proportion of the total medicines market accounted for by fake products typically range from around 10% to in the order of 20 or 30%. Significant numbers of (in particular poor) people suffer harm as a result of this trade, which can in part be seen as a symptom of other forms of corruption and imperfection in healthcare markets. Ensuring the integrity (as well as the equity) of global medicines supply should be seen as an international priority for the early 21st century.
2. Historically, western Europe has enjoyed a well-regulated

and secure pharmaceutical market. In the 1980s and 1990s there were far fewer reported cases of medicine counterfeiting reported in the 'old EU' than in the USA. Yet this should not be taken as a justification for complacency. Europe is changing, and more cases of fake medicine supply are being reported.

3 The international record shows that counterfeiting risks arise from many factors. In Europe practices such as parallel importing and generic medicines use should not be unfairly blamed for being a root cause of criminal behaviour. But there is good reason to argue that they have served to undermine medicines supply chain security, in ways that may eventually come to be seen as seriously damaging.

With regard to the last point, it can also be suggested that just as traders in pharmaceutical parallel imports should not be wrongly accused of illicit behaviour, Europeans and their political leaders should be careful not to unfairly vilify research-based pharmaceutical companies. At times such organisations appear irrationally to be held responsible for problems well outside their actual ambit of control. These range from the inadequate provision of international (pharmaceutical) aid to the world's poorest communities to the rising costs of healthcare among its most affluent populations.

Given Europe's long-term interest in retaining research-based enterprise and maintaining its populations' standard of living, developing a balanced and constructive overall set of EU pharmaceutical sector policies is an important priority. So too is developing better community-wide understanding of issues relating to the funding and practical achievement of biomedical innovation, such as balancing desires for increased drug safety with those for finding more effective treatments for conditions such as cancers, rheumatic diseases and neurological disorders such as multiple sclerosis and the dementias.

The recent establishment of a European Union Pharmaceutical Forum, intended to improve the EU's pharmaceutical sector competitiveness, may prove a significant step in this direction. Its primary areas of interest are Health Technology Assessment (HTA – in particular focused on evaluating the comparative efficacy and effectiveness of new and established treatments), the impacts of Europe's complex pharmaceutical price controls, and the accessibility to the public of medicines and other health-related information.

From the perspective of this chapter and the growing awareness of the threat that medicines counterfeiting presents, however, additional questions that the Forum's members may wish to research include:

- Will an expanded and more diverse Europe be able to maintain pharmaceutical supply chain integrity in an affordable, cost-effective manner? Exploring this area should arguably require an open, publicly transparent risk analysis, conducted to a standard equivalent to that employed in assessing biomedical risk during licensing assessments.
- What are the total costs and benefits of medicines parallel importing in the EU? This could include an evaluation of all direct, indirect and intangible regulatory and PI medicine supply costs (incorporating factors such as the diversion of professional pharmacy time into 'cheap'

medicines purchasing and as and when it occurs patient confusion resulting from unfamiliar presentations being supplied) and an analysis of this trade's total impact on the research-based pharmaceutical industry in Europe and elsewhere. Costs may include not only research funding problems, but those of managerial attempts to moderate the effects of parallel trade on medicine patent holders' revenue streams.

- How should the European Union and/or Europe more widely seek to minimise the future harm associated with medicines counterfeiting? If it were concluded that removing incentives for parallel trading would be desirable on public health or other grounds the Forum's work on pharmaceutical pricing should in part focus on identifying how to deliver any public-interest-related benefits of the current pattern of parallel importing, without its unwanted aspects.
- What could US and other policy-makers learn from the EU's experience with pharmaceutical parallel importing, and what should EU decision-makers learn from the experiences of countries such as the USA, India, China and Nigeria in the context of trading in fake medicines?

From a European viewpoint it is relevant to note that the US pharmaceutical market has grown in value much faster than the EU's since the beginning of the 1990s. Notwithstanding currency adjustments, it can reasonably be estimated that American medicine users now fund some 50% (by cost) of all medicines research conducted worldwide. At the same time India and China are moving rapidly to extend their capacities in this area. They have the advantage of a large, increasingly educated yet still low-cost labour force, anxious to advance in the world.

Some US policy-makers believe that radical reductions in US medicine costs could be achieved by allowing on a commercial basis the reimportation of patent-protected American and other pharmaceutical innovations into the US market from regions such as the EU and Canada, where state controls require relatively low prices. One effect of this, however, would be to reduce the funding available to American companies to invest in Europe-based research laboratories and other facilities. From an American position it might also be seen as a surrender of sovereignty, in that it would in effect allow foreign market interventions into the US domestic economy. That is, it would in effect bypass US policies on pricing and allied market freedoms. In addition, it could further complicate the task of the FDA and other agencies seeking to protect the quality of US medicines.

Conclusion

The basic answer to the question *'What could and should European stakeholders in safe medicines supply be doing about medicines counterfeiting?'* is that they should stop denying the reality of the threat it represents, and take it seriously.

European public interests in pharmaceutical development and use are complex. Oversimplified arguments that imply that cost minimisation is always in taxpayers' or other healthcare funders' interests should not be uncritically accepted, and the significance of findings such as those of the Council of Europe on the scale and threat of medicines counterfeiting in modern Europe should be recognised in as honest and objective a manner as possible. The part that practices such as parallel importing may play in increasing risks should not be minimised because – for example – national-level officials believe (almost certainly wrongly) that the expenditure savings it generates fund – or at least legitimise – their jobs.

Were a counterfeiting episode to be seen to kill a significant number of patients, it would harm the credibility and standing of all the agencies involved, from the European Commission and member state regulators and policy-makers to the pharmaceutical industry and the profession of pharmacy. Awareness of this fact, coupled with the fundamentally important concern of people in civilised communities to go on improving public health and protecting individual citizens from avoidable harm, will hopefully be sufficient to promote a sense of common interest in combating medicines counterfeiting in Europe. The realisation of this goal in practice will demand effective reform, aimed at rebuilding and where possible enhancing the integrity of the European medicines supply chain.

3

Finding common ground: policy imperatives for Europe[1]

Michael Tremblay

Counterfeiting is about patient safety

The problem of medicines counterfeiting is usually seen as a problem with theft of intellectual property rights, making the issue one little different from copying music CDs or movie DVDs, or even fake designer jeans. But it is increasingly obvious that there is no consensus on what the real problem of medicines counterfeiting is.

The pharmaceutical industry and existing legislation view the problem in terms of intellectual property, while police and customs officials see the issue as one of criminal activity or illegal trade. There is rising concern that organised crime and terrorist groups are interested in the counterfeiting of medicines (Satchwell, 2004).

This diversity of opinion in terms of what the problem is

makes counterfeiting more complex, reflecting these differing notions of what the solution should be. If we are not clear as to what the problem is, of course, then we may pursue solutions that do not, in the end, solve it. Regardless of whether these different opinions have separate merit, the problem of counterfeiting, by virtue of a lack of consensus on what the real problem is, risks being little understood – this has the added disbenefit of ensuring that any data we do have may not help us understand the problem. By advocating different positions, well-intentioned thinking simplifies the problem in such a way as to leave unsolved the specific concerns that others have.

When complex systems misbehave, they may do so because designers have inadequately or incompletely specified what rules (laws, procedures, protocols, etc.) should govern the system, or because others are exploiting weaknesses in the system. On the other hand, people are wont to treat complexity as a combination of simple elements, each of which can be understood, while largely ignoring that more complex interconnectivity (Rittel, 1972; Rittel and Webber, 1973, 1984).

Complicating the problem of counterfeiting is its international nature, and what happens when one country's system of medicines regulation or law enforcement has to interact with another country's to deal with a counterfeit medicine. This is where we discover that there are gaps in regulations between countries caused by differing notions of what counterfeiting is, different enforcement practices, even different definitions of what counterfeit medicines are. But one country's regulatory system cannot have influence outside that country, so to overcome this international treaties are developed to express common intent, to define the realm of shared action and regularise inter-state relations.

While counterfeiting involves intellectual property, organised crime and a whole raft of other concerns, it is essentially a problem that exploits weaknesses within a *designed system* of medicines manufacture, shipping, prescribing and dispensing, involving a vast array of potentially disorganised and disconnected organisations, companies, governments and regulators – a designed system concerned with delivering safe medicines from manufacturer to patient. But how many fatalities are needed before safety becomes the focus of attention of this system?[2]

To date, coherent international action to address the threat of counterfeiting has been absent. This may be changing, though, and progress towards coordinated international action may be forthcoming following the WHO conference in Rome specifically focused on this issue in February 2005 (WHO, 2006). International concerted action must also work from a common understanding of the problem, however, defined through shared definitions and priorities.

We need to treat counterfeit medicines as what they are, a clear and present threat to human health – and to *patient safety*. This simplifies much of the debate, providing a common framework for action by all interested groups, and more clearly identifying what needs to be done.

Regulatory denial

Within the spectrum of interests, special attention must be paid to national medicines regulators. Regretfully, much medicines regulation focuses on regulating the medicines themselves, and documenting approval of companies to engage in the medicines trade. This means that systemic problems that cut across the regulatory rules may fail to register as priorities because they fall outside the regulator's formal jurisdiction, and may be a concern for industry or another regulatory body or agency. A simple example involves distinguishing between the regulator's licensing of companies to import medicines, and national customs enforcement of importation: the former enables the latter to act, while the latter is responsible for detecting criminal conduct by those licensed by the former. A third body may be required to enforce regulatory compliance, and a fourth may deal with recovery of payment for the medicines. In the meantime, commercial partners in the pharmaceutical supply chain continue to be confronted with rogue traders and must improvise their own disparate solutions.

This means that regulators are often prevented by their mandates from acting on suspicions that there may be threats to the security of the medicine supply chain from counterfeit medicines which arise from the jurisdictional failures of other bodies. As well, enforcement bodies are often prevented from proactively raising the profile of failures in policy or weaknesses in law that create these opportunities for counterfeiters in the first place, if they construe their enforcement mandate narrowly – in other words, if the country does not prioritise counterfeiting, then why should the police?

This regulatory denial is unhelpful with problems that are emergent and in the early stages of becoming major. And this denial is reinforced when concerted action across borders is required and international agreements are lacking. In Europe, the situation is complicated by the requirements of the single market, the open border with free movement of goods, and where existing European Union (EU) medicines regulation fails to adequately frame counterfeiting in a EU context. A similar situation exists between Canada and the USA.

The absence of comprehensive and reliable data on the prevalence of counterfeit drugs also means that regulators, rightly from their perspective, can say there really is no major problem. Lacking good information makes it more difficult to justify raising the priority of counterfeiting. That there have been no major scandals and health catastrophes in any European member state is taken by regulators as evidence that the system is working; the situation is no different in other countries where discussion on counterfeiting is muted. And so the denial is reinforced by whatever poor-quality empirical evidence exists. This, in turn, does not justify urgent action by law-makers.

But more than that, poor data undermine proper understanding of the potential scope of the global medicines counterfeiting 'industry' itself. The failure to pool information and knowledge and adopt common definitions and data means that differences between national regulators will continue to frustrate a coherent response to the problem at an EU or international level.

The way regulators enforce the rules is also relevant in terms of how effective any system of vigilance and reporting can be (Walshe, 2003). Punitive systems are unlikely to encourage pharmacists to come forward with evidence of counterfeits for fear that their licences may be suspended pending an investigation. Unsophisticated policing may compound the problem by pursuing investigations ineffectively, while the public is kept in the dark by official silence on the part of all concerned. Safety is not enhanced when honest people live in fear of punishment.

This lack of consensus among regulators means that driving forward inter-state regulatory convergence on enforcement, cross-border exchange of information and coordinated detection and enforcement will be very difficult to achieve.

It may be easier to add 'soft law' approaches to dealing with counterfeit medicines, using inter-sectoral collaboration with actors who operate across borders, as governments will encounter more difficulties seeking to extend jurisdiction; leadership from industry, for instance, with government policy and legislative support, offers one approach that is compatible with approaches to international safety from other sectors.

Public confidence has yet to be shaken

A frequent observation within the EU, the USA, Canada and other major countries has concerned the relatively little evidence of significant numbers of counterfeit drugs in these countries. This is to be contrasted with their presence in quantity in many developing countries.

There are many reasons why this may be the case, although, as has been noted, regulators would argue that superior regulation is the main reason. We know that the number of cases of counterfeit medicines is rising in the USA, however, and an increased incidence in the EU is evidence of weaknesses in cross-border medicines regulation, which may be emboldening counterfeiters.

What is important, though, is that just because no event of signficance has taken place in the EU, this should not be seen as justifying complacency. Indeed, what would count as evidence of a significant event? There is concern that some anecdotal incidences of adverse reactions to medicines may arise from the presence of counterfeits, but we have no evidence since adverse reactions to medicines rarely if ever lead to examination of the medicine itself. There is also speculation that some instances of patient death may have been hastened by counterfeit medicines,[3] but it is hard to prove that a counterfeit medicine actually *caused* death, especially with patients who are already in a weakened state of health.

Regardless of our position on the reliability of empirical evidence to the contrary, people take their medicines because they trust the safety of the medicine, they trust the pharmacist and they trust their prescriber – they trust the system. Loss of public trust in the safety of medicines is inconceivable given the way the prescribing system works. The consequences of public distrust would have significant consequences for the regulation, manufacture, packaging, supply and dispensing of medicine.

Fortunately, we can take heart that a proactive response in the absence of compelling evidence is not irrational because we can invoke the so-called 'precautionary principle', which states: *When an activity raises threats of harm to human health or the environment, precautionary measures should be taken even if some cause-and-effect relationships are not fully established scientifically* (Tickner et al., 1998).

What this says to us as we think about how to deal with counterfeit medicines is that we need to do two things:

- *think ahead*: do not wait for problems to become fully evident before collecting information, thinking about solutions, improving regulation, protecting the supply chain, engaging with the public about good medicines practices; and

- *act before there is a crisis*: delay will only give the counterfeiters additional time to consolidate their actions, conceal their methods and develop further sophistication in frustrating detection.

Failure here will only create a situation in which governments, industry and regulators will need to act out of urgency in responding to heightened public anxiety, but citizens are not well served when governments engage in hasty law-making, behaving in an authoritarian manner to produce poor-quality laws and regulations.

We can never be complacent about standards of safety and security, and these simple requirements, coupled with concerted and shared EU and international action, are the best ways forward.

The pharmaceutical safety chain[5]

If we accept that the problem of counterfeiting is really a patient safety problem, we have the opportunity to think about what sort of system or approach can best define the necessary common ground.

In other sectors, safety improvement is linked to the use of a *safety chain*, to enable inter-sectoral collaboration; with medicines we have governments, regulators, pharmaceutical manufacturers, wholesalers, distributors, health purchasers, healthcare professionals and patients, who all need to be brought together.

The 'pharmaceutical safety chain' provides an integrated and *interlocking* approach to safety by creating expectations, responsibilities and accountabilities that define safety priorities and responses. Drawing on lessons from maritime, food, banking and agricultural industries, the pharmaceutical safety chain represents a state-of-the-art approach to inter-sector safety improvement to eliminate the presence of counterfeit medicines.

As we have argued, counterfeit medicines present a patient safety threat, and safety is a shared responsibility. Therefore, a collaborative approach is necessary to identify and solve safety problems. The safety chain approach, using standards, track-and-trace technologies and uniform event reporting, provides higher standards of safety and security through a system of interlocking obligations between actors across the supply chain. This requires supply chain actors to verify that both the origin of the medicine they are purchasing or handling and its next destination involve organisations that adhere to standards of a 'pharmaceutical trade safety chain', which is defined as *a voluntary assurance system embracing everyone involved in the trade of medicines to enable consistent safety practice through high standards and the transparent exchange of information from surveillance and monitoring of trading practices, to support and enhance public confidence.*

Information on the movement of medicines would be collected using appropriate technologies and disseminated to support compliance and trading transparency. Standards will be developed and adhered to by the groups participating in the safety chain.

Benefits of a safety chain

A safety chain directly addresses the counterfeiting of medicines. Specifically:

It should be easier to identify non-conforming or non-participating organisations, or weak regulatory regimes, to determine whether non-compliance is a form of evasion or failure to meet agreed standards.

1. The safety chain makes it easier to identify and remedy risky or non-compliant trading activities that create incentives for counterfeiters.
2. Purchasers of products at any stage of the supply chain can expect suppliers to meet the obligations of safety chain practices and standards, and vice versa.
3. It captures information on the movement of medicines and makes it easier to track and trace products.
4. An electronic database, forming the spine of the safety chain, would provide seamless information to support safety chain activities, support transparency and enable greater accountability.

In addition, implementation of a safety chain will necessitate review of a range of existing legislation to ensure that there are no perverse 'incentives' contributing to the counterfeiting problem.

Europe needs a cross-border solution

The European Union presents a particularly complex environment for dealing with the threat from counterfeit medicines.

The single market rules protect the free movement of goods across the internal borders of the EU. In addition, unlike the FDA (Food and Drug Administration) in the USA, EMEA (European Medicines Evaluation Agency) is not the EU regulator with competency to deal with counterfeits, as individual member state medicines regulators have this responsibility. There is a large body of European Union legislation[5] that is relevant to pharmaceutical products, including directives that enhance EU oversight of manufacturing so that it complies with GMP guidance.

But the European Union system is best understood as a devolved and uncoordinated system, lacking EU-wide enforcement, effective and timely alerting systems and a comprehensive collection of information.

The elimination of internal border controls means that counterfeit products move within the provisions of single-market rules, which weakens cross-border detection of counterfeits. Member states lack the authority to take regulatory action against suppliers in other member states. The porosity of the EU's external border to entry of counterfeit medicines from traders who exploit the different weaknesses in member state border controls only highlights the need for consistent policing of the external frontier.

Despite the best intentions of EMEA and the European Commission, there are differences in how individual member state medicines regulators undertake their work, as well as in how different countries have organised their national medicines supply chains. These inconsistencies become potential weaknesses when seen at an international level, but they are particularly troublesome within the EU, where inter-state differences are not supposed to significantly influence trade between member states and where a consistent environment of rules should prevail.

The Treaty of Rome stipulations that bestow on member states control over their health systems[6] appear to have been extended to include oversight of the pharmaceutical industry and its products through national pricing controls. It is open to some question, however, as to whether pricing control of medicines by national authorities is compatible within the context of the EU as a whole.[7] Certainly, the marketing authorisations, which do fall within member state competence and are perhaps compatible with their authority to protect human health, should not be confused with subsequent pricing policies by these same member states. Indeed, it may be that these pricing policies, as a price divergence between member states, create exploitable opportunities for trade in counterfeit medicines.

This is comparable to the situation in the United States, and may be incentivising counterfeiters and rogue traders to exploit these price differentials (Eban, 2005).

The lack of a single market in medicines encourages specific forms of EU cross-border trade, but the state-based regulation means that repackaging, and other requirements to meet national market features, creates vulnerabilities in the supply chain, which can be exploited for criminal gain.

In addition, the approach taken by current EU legislation assigns priority to the intellectual property rights of trademark holders, and views this as providing appropriate protection against counterfeits.[8] The patient safety issue thereby falls to member state authorities.

European Union and international priorities: an agenda for action

The EU needs to define a collective response to address current deficiencies and move forward with a coherent policy, and a legislative response to counterfeit medicines. This agenda will require action by the Council on the inter-governmental priorities, by the European Commission for specific EU priorities, and by the European Parliament on behalf of European citizens.

A four-point programme of action is proposed comprising:

1. a consistent policy environment to tackle counterfeiting at the EU level;
2. a legislative and regulatory review of EU and member states rules, and regulations;
3. research to quantify the current state of counterfeiting;
4. improved security of the supply chain at the EU level.

Create a consistent policy environment at the EU level

Patient safety is an EU and cross-border priority.[9] Given the considerable impact counterfeit drugs can have on human health, patient safety should be established as the over-arching rationale for acting on counterfeits. The 'pharmaceutical safety chain' can be used as the basic framework to create the necessary consistency of action among all the social partners.

The Rome WHO conference on counterfeit medicines has identified a direction for concerted international action. In light of that, a review of future legislative direction with the European Union should be undertaken looking at all areas relevant to counterfeit medicines, with a view to establishing consistency in going forward.

Conduct a legislative and regulatory review

The freedom of movement of medicines within the EU may create incentives that make it difficult to track and identify counterfeit products and rogue traders of counterfeit medicines; accordingly, a review of the single-market rules is called for, covering EU and member state areas of competency, to assess this.

Given evidence from other jurisdictions, a review of the drug reimbursement policies of member states is needed to determine whether member-state control of medicines pricing and the resulting price divergence create an incentive for counterfeiters and their trading partners to exploit price differentials through the parallel trade in medicines within the EU.

The legislative review should determine whether there are unintended consequences arising from existing legislation and incompatibilities in existing legislation that may restrict or inhibit the ability of key groups to be able to communicate information to the public about counterfeit medicines and risks to health; this would be relevant to governments as well as to companies, NGOs and patient groups, and should address in particular the provisions of the Advertising Directive[10] and transposing legislation in the member states.

The different practices of the EU member states need to be 'mapped' to identify where mismatches in regulatory practices may contribute to problems at the EU level or between the member states themselves; this 'cross-border regulatory map' should identify how enforcement practices differ, and consider inconsistencies in terms of definitions of counterfeiting and data collection practices. The benchmarking of regulatory performance should also be undertaken as part of this to provide the basis for consistent and high standards in going forward.

Quantify the current state of counterfeiting in the EU

Research could be commissioned on the extent and nature of counterfeiting within the EU. The Council of Europe research[11] has shown that there really is a knowledge gap in our ability to quantify the scale of medicines counterfeiting. We need to know how counterfeit products enter the EU and how they move between member states. We also need to know how effectively member states police the external EU border to identify counterfeit medicines at the point of entry.

Improve the security of the supply chain at the EU level

The 'pharmaceutical safety chain' approach identifies a way to improve supply chain security to ensure patient safety. Working from that basis, a variety of areas need inter-sectoral attention (at the EU and member state levels, in industry and among patient groups and technology partners) to bring a heightened level of security to the medicines supply chain.

Action is appropriate in the following areas:

- Standards of security and safety are needed that reflect the fact that the EU supply chain is not secure in the presence of counterfeits and the actions of rogue traders.
- Good data collection, analysis and monitoring are needed to inform policy-makers, regulators, industry and the

public to ensure a high level of understanding of safety across the EU supply chain.
- Ways to adopt technologies to achieve track-and-trace capabilities across the EU supply chain need to be identified.

To improve sharing of information between regulators, the EU should have a central clearing house of information on all companies and organisations involved in the movement of medicines within, across, into and out of the EU, and which provides access to member-state regulatory documents and licences from any of the member-state jurisdictions; standard formats and information should prevail to meet the diverse needs of users in other member states.

Concluding remarks

Counterfeiting is a complex patient safety problem with a solution that must engage all social partners, from government and regulators to industry and patients, in finding common ground to move forward with a shared solution. Internationally, there is clearly much work that needs to be done. This chapter has laid out the agenda for specific action by the European Union and its member states.

Technical appendix on the pharmaceutical safety chain

The structure of the pharmaceutical safety chain

The figure and table below illustrate the key elements of the

SAFETY TOOLS	SAFETY ACTIONS				
	PRO-ACTION	PREVENTION	PREPARATION	MITIGATION	RECOVERY
PLANNING	Develop safety model	Understand stakeholder needs	Develop responses	Plan for threats	Learn the lessons from incidents
STANDARDS	Define standards	*EU wide coding standards*		Review and improve standards	Produce revised standards
DATABASE	Information reporting, alerts	*Shared database*			
CODING	Agree coding technologies	*Information collection*			
IMPLEMENTATION	Collaborative approach	*Quality Assurance System*	*Build response capabilities*	*Standards of practice*	Solve the counterfeiting problem

Figure 3 **Responsibilities of safety chain actors**

safety chain, along with identified responsibilities and associated actions for actors.

Definitions

Key steps in the safety chain are adapted from those used in civil protection,[12] comprising a comprehensive framework covering planning about safety and the prevention of accidents, preparations for responding to incidents, and the mitigation of the consequences of safety-related incidents, as well as ways of learning from the experience and implementing changes to maintain a high standard of safety. The key activities are:

Table 1 The groups comprising the links in the safety chain

Group	*Originators of medicines*	*Licensed trading companies including final purchasers of medicines*	*Governments and regulators*	*Dispensers of medicines*	*End-users*
Definition	Manufacturers of medicines	Firms that operate between manufacturers and end-users, to move products through the supply chain, comprising wholesalers, shippers, redistributors and parallel traders; included here are state or public purchasers and their national distribution systems	Bodies that are concerned with the legal or regulatory aspects of trade in medicines and human health	Those who dispense, and are the last step before the patient, comprising pharmacists in hospital or community, dispensing doctors, hospital specialists	These are patients, parents, informal carers and consumers, as well as non-dispensing prescribers
Safety interests and priorities	Integrity of the manufactured medicinal product Safety of the medicine	Control of the logistics process and movement of the actual product Quality and value for money	Public safety and public health Legal and regulatory compliance	Mitigation of product-related risk Customer service and quality	Product quality Trust in the safe supply of medicines

Proaction

Safety standards are needed along with consensus on information requirements including agreement on an appropriate technology platform to support coding. Consensus is also needed on day-to-day operations and links with existing practice.

Prevention

The safety needs of everyone in the supply chain must involve shared understanding. Central to identification of counterfeiting in particular is an over-arching single responsible body, similar to organisations in other industries (for example, the International Maritime Organisation).

Preparation

Everyone needs to build response capabilities to assure the public that appropriate steps are being taken.

Mitigation

The development of interventions to manage incidents of counterfeiting is a shared responsibility, with methods to be agreed.

Recovery

Everyone must learn from mistakes and accidents, and take appropriate steps to reform practice, and revise standards.

To implement these various activities, we need specific tools and techniques. All the most effective safety chains studied utilised in some form or other these key tools. Overall, these will require a 'technology platform' to enable the database and coding.

Planning

Agreement by everyone on the values, purpose and design of the safety system to detect counterfeits. This will require discussion and development, plus a continuing commitment to safety, through a shared forward-planning framework.

Standards

The safety chain depends on agreement and application of standards covering trading practices, types of information required, reporting requirements and regulatory practice. These would apply nationally and crucially across borders to track products and identify counterfeits.

Database

All the safety-related information, including that involving flagging up problems, reviewing problems, and supporting regulatory and trading standards compliance, needs to be organised.

Coding

A consistent approach to data elements is needed to support the ability of the database to inform the standards, and to support implementation and compliance.

Implementation

A single organisation may be needed to take over-arching and EU or international responsibility for ensuring the quality of the standards, to receive the information from the coding, to house the database, and to report on compliance. This body should also respond to public enquiries.

Background to the development of the safety chain concept

The development of a safety chain to deal with medicines counterfeiting draws on thinking carried out in other sectors. A safety chain oversees maritime shipping, bringing together governments, insurers, shipowners and port authorities.[13] Food

Table 2 Lessons on safety for the pharmaceutical industry from other industries

Area	*Feature*	*Design lesson for counterfeiting*
Banking	Cheque-clearing system and security Fraud and counterfeiting	Ensure security of processes, including knowing identity of sources and destinations of medicines
Auto racing	Inherently dangerous Manage and control risk	Some things are in fact dangerous; in some cases risk needs to be managed, and danger is unavoidable
Airlines	Design to eliminate risk as much as possible	Identify areas of risk and danger to the public and work to eliminate the risk as much as possible
Food	Provenance 'food safety chain' links public health, animal health, plant health and the environment Due diligence between buyers and sellers	Formal links between different actors, with mutual expectations and checking of compliance using track-and-traceability technology and flow of information to monitor shipments of medicines and identify rogue shipments
Environmental protection	Precautionary principle	Counterfeiting may be an area where action is needed before there is sufficient evidence
Shipping	Maritime safety chain	Each party has defined and shared areas of responsibility Clear focus on addressing problems of non-compliance by the 'weak links'
Civil protection	Population-based risk	Proactive approach that integrates both actors and processes, focused on patient safety and counterfeiting

safety in the UK is governed by a chain linking retail outlets, farmers and food processors and packers, and with track-and-traceability requirements to ensure food provenance with a duty of 'due diligence' among supply-chain actors.[14] Many countries already use 'chain of custody'-type thinking to ensure appropriate linkages between actors working together.

Highlights of the safety lessons from other sectors are summarised in Table 2.

In addition, thinking about safety itself was guided by the Institute of Medicine's *To Err Is Human* (IoM, 2000), and its key principles for safety:

1. the need for leadership to deal with the problem of counterfeiting;
2. the development of simple, transparent, understandable whole-system processes;
3. team working, rather than silos of accountability, appropriate to the cross-jurisdictional nature of safety with the need for shared learning and without imposed solutions;
4. being proactive, rather than waiting for a crisis to justify action;
5. fostering a learning environment, based on training, research and standards, recognising that safety is a complex, multi-dimensional, cross-jurisdictional issue requiring iterative learning.

4

Counterfeit medicines in less developed countries: problems and solutions

Julian Morris and Philip Stevens

Much of the debate surrounding counterfeit medicines to date has focused on how to prevent them seeping into the supply chains of developed-country markets. The majority of counterfeit medicines originate in Less Developed Countries (LDCs), including most of those that end up in the USA and the EU. Steps should be taken to change the incentives faced by counterfeiters in LDCs to participate in the production and trade of counterfeit pharmaceuticals.

The scale of the problem

While counterfeit medicines in wealthy markets are a growing concern for physicians and law enforcement agencies, their prevalence pales in comparison to their penetration of less developed markets. According to the World Health Organisation (WHO), 25% of all medicines in LDCs are counterfeit.[1] In some countries, the prevalence is far higher:

- Counterfeit medicines constitute between 40% and 50% of total supply in Nigeria and Pakistan (Gibson, 2004).
- In China, authorities have found that some products have a counterfeit prevalence ranging between 50% and 85%.[2]
- 36.5% of antibiotics and anti-malarials on the WHO essential drugs list in Thailand and Nigeria are sub-standard (Shakoor et al., 1997).
- A recent survey by the WHO of seven African countries found that between 20% and 90% of all anti-malarials failed quality testing. These included chloroquine-based syrup and tablets, whose failure rate ranged from 23% to 38%; and sulphadoxine/pyrimethamine tablets, up to 90% of which were found to be below standard (WHO, 2003).

In spite of a lack of hard data (Cockburn et al., 2005), it is clear that counterfeit medicines are not confined to a handful of therapeutic classes. This is especially true in LDCs, where the range of fakes on the markets encompasses treatments for a diverse range of conditions and ailments. The top five counterfeited medicines in the Philippines provide some illustration of this point:

1. Anti-hypertensive drugs (Adalat Gits 30mg tablet)
2. Anti-asthma drugs (Ventolin expectorant syrup)
3. Analgesic medicines (Ponstan 500)
4. Anti-diarrhoea (Diatabs reformulated)
5. Vitamins (Propan with iron capsule, Ceelin 100 mg/5 ml syrup, Enervon C and Iberet 500)[3]

This list is certainly not exhaustive. Other favourites for counterfeiting include drugs for treating anaemia, HIV and schizophrenia, as well as growth promotion hormone (used in the treatment of HIV). The problem also extends beyond fake pharmaceuticals to medical consumables such as non-sterile syringes and gauze, and even sub-standard electronic medical equipment.

Where are counterfeit medicines being produced?

A large proportion of the world's counterfeit medicines originate in Asia. China in particular is a production centre, although precise data about the scale and scope of the problem within this country are neither widely available nor reliable. In 2001 it was reported that China had 500 illegal medicines factories, and while no newer data are available, it is safe to assume that number has since increased.[4] Also in 2001, it was reported that Chinese authorities 'closed 1,300 factories while investigating 480,000 cases of counterfeit drugs worth $57 million' (Fackler, 2002). Most Chinese counterfeit medicines that find their way into foreign supply chains first pass through the ports of Hong Kong and Shenzhen.

South-East Asia more generally is a major source of counterfeit medicines. According to the WHO, Cambodia had 2,800 illegal medicine sellers and 1,000 unregistered drugs on the market in 2003. The same report showed that Laos had about 2,100 illegal medicines sellers, while in Thailand sub-standard medicines account for approximately 8.5% of the total market.[5]

One 2002 study by government officials showed that 9% of all drugs tested in *India* were sub-standard.[6] Some 15,000 generics manufacturers operate in India.[7] Although the majority are legitimate, a small minority are likely to be 'fly by night' operations that do not comply with proper standards. Most of the counterfeit medicines in *Nigeria* originate in India, a fact that led the Nigerian authorities to threaten to ban the import of all drugs from India in 2003 (Raufu, 2003). It should be noted, however, that 70% of the Indian domestic market is supplied by around twenty companies that regularly pass inspections from visiting officials from Western countries.[8]

Counterfeit medicines also abound in *Latin America*, with instances reported in Argentina, Brazil, Colombia, Venezuela, Mexico, Peru and Guatemala: *Mexico* is a major global source of counterfeit medicines, with the trade standing at an estimated value of US$650 million per year – equal to around 10% of total drug sales in the country.[9]

In *Russia*, it is estimated that counterfeits constitute between 5% and 10% of the total market.[10] In 1999 alone, 1,500 lots of Russian-made drugs failed to pass quality tests.[11]

The impact of counterfeit medicines

Counterfeit medicines can cause harm in various ways: the presence of toxic chemicals frequently causes injury or death; inappropriate delivery systems and/or inadequate amounts of active ingredient prevent the drugs from working effectively and, again, can lead to injury or death; more broadly, under-dosing fosters resistance to the active chemical. In the cases of HIV/Aids and malaria, this latter aspect is particularly worrying.

Harm

Counterfeit medicines often contain agents that are injurious to health, as, for example, when 89 people in Haiti died after ingesting cough syrup manufactured with diethylene glycol (a chemical commonly used as antifreeze). This particular product was made in China and transported through a Dutch company to Germany, before winding up on the Haitian market. A similar case occurred in Nigeria in 1995, resulting in the death of 109 children, and again in Bangladesh (Hanif et al., 1995).

The dangers of widespread counterfeiting were illustrated in 1996 during a meningitis epidemic in Nigeria. Some 60,000 people were inoculated with counterfeit vaccines, resulting in the deaths of 2,500 people (Pécoul et al., 1999).

More importantly, counterfeit medicines typically provide inadequate doses of drugs, either because too little active ingredient is included in pills or because the delivery vehicle (including otherwise 'inactive' ingredients) is inappropriate (for example, chemicals that are not water-soluble). As a result, patients receive too little medicine and die or are far sicker than would have been the case if they had received an adequate dose.

It is estimated that in China between 200,000 and 300,000 people die each year owing to counterfeit or sub-standard medicine. However, this 'official' statistic may over- or understate the true number of cases. And these are reported cases: the true number of cases is likely to be far higher.[12]

Drug resistance

Perhaps one of the most worrying implications of the global boom in counterfeit medicines is the acceleration of new, drug-resistant strains of viruses, parasites and bacteria. If drugs contain too little of the active ingredient, not all the disease agents are killed and resistant strains are able to multiply and spread.

Malaria

This is already being observed in the treatment of malaria. Counterfeiters around the world have cashed in on the massive demand for the latest and most effective anti-malarial drug, artemisinin. A field survey conducted in 2004 showed that 53% of artemisinin-based anti-malarials in a range of South-East Asian countries contained incorrect levels of active ingredient (Dondorp et al., 2004), which implies that swaths of patients are receiving the incorrect dose. The direct consequences are death and serious injury resulting from improper treatment.

In addition, exposing malaria parasites to inadequate (sub-therapeutic) concentrations of artesunate may result in the multiplication of parasites resistant to the drug (White, 1999). Even though artemisinin has been widely available only since the late 1990s, scientists are already reporting cases of resistance. According to Dr Dora Akunyili, the head of Nigeria's national drug regulator, the racket in fake medicine is directly responsible for this resistance, and is a contributing factor to the doubling of malaria deaths over the last twenty years.[13]

HIV/AIDS

HIV/AIDS treatment is also under threat from counterfeit medicines. The recent discovery of counterfeit anti-retrovirals (stavudine-lamivudine-nevirapine and lamivudine-zidovudine) in the Congo (Ahmad, 2004) raises the prospect that the first-line therapies for the treatment of HIV/AIDS could soon be rendered useless. With few new research leads in the pipeline, this could have grave implications for the people of sub-Saharan Africa.

Bird flu

Finally, counterfeit medicines could be undermining our ability to contain and treat a potential avian flu pandemic. As demand has grown for the anti-viral drug Tamiflu, one of the best current treatments for the disease, counterfeiters have ramped up production of illegitimate versions. Already, the Internet is awash with spurious Tamiflu, while consignments have been discovered as far apart as New York and Beijing. The risk is that copies containing sub-therapeutic levels of active ingredient could facilitate the development of drug-resistant forms of the avian flu virus, leaving very few tools to contain a potential pandemic.

Undermining R&D

Counterfeiting can also undermine the incentives of R&D-based companies to invest in future innovation. Even near-perfect copies of non-patent medicines cause harm by competing with legitimate supplies of medicines from originating companies, which reduces revenues and undermines incentives to invest in future R&D.

Underlying causes of LDC counterfeiting

- **Absent or defective IP protection.** One way to prevent the sale of unauthorised copies of medicines is to enable companies to register and enforce trademarks. These enable vendors to signal the quality of their product to potential purchasers. Trademark owners have strong incentives to ensure that the quality of their product is maintained because their reputation and hence future profitability depend upon it. In many LDCs it is difficult to enforce trademarks – even for local companies. Where trademarks cannot be enforced, cheaply produced poor-quality copies will typically crowd out good-quality drugs.

- **Lack of adequate civil liability.** Civil law protects the consumer against missold or defective goods. By enabling consumers (or their relatives) to obtain redress from the manufacturer or supplier of a harmful product, such liability both compensates those who are harmed and discourages manufacturers and suppliers from selling counterfeits. In many LDCs, however, civil law is either poorly defined or difficult to enforce.
- **Inability to resolve disputes over property rights and contracts in independent courts.** Underlying the lack of civil liability and weak IP protection are dysfunctional and inefficient legal systems. As a result, it can often take years for cases to be heard. Many courts in LDCs are hampered by inefficient processes, causing delays. In many LDCs law enforcement is also corrupt. In such places, criminal counterfeiting gangs may be able to pay corrupt law enforcement agents to turn a blind eye to their activities. If a case does make it to court, the gangs may be able to pay off the judge and thereby induce a favourable judgment.
- **Weak or absent rule of law.** In LDCs with a weak rule of law, political and legal decisions tend to be arbitrary and

designed to benefit the elite. As a result, regulation designed to combat counterfeiting is often ineffective. Corruption within regulatory agencies and police forces exacerbates this problem, so that the enforcement of regulations is seen as an opportunity to collect bribes.

- **Price controls.** The imposition of price controls by governments prevents companies from selling goods at different prices to different consumers. Also, where prices are controlled at different levels in different markets, traders exploit these price differentials through arbitrage. Such trade (called parallel trade) may create gaps in the supply chain which can be exploited by counterfeiters. For example, it is often necessary to repackage drugs in order to sell them in a different market, which requires re-labelling in the correct language. This creates opportunities for unscrupulous intermediaries to infiltrate the supply chain with fakes. Price controls in wealthy country markets therefore increase the chance that copies of patented medicines produced in LDCs will leak back into wealthy-country markets. In addition, companies have less incentive to register products in markets where their drugs are subject to price controls, leading to shortages in supplies. They also reduce the margins made by pharmacies, making the distribution of drugs to remote and rural regions financially unviable. For example, the price caps forced on certain drugs in South Africa have been implicated in the closure of 103 pharmacies.[14] If markets are left unsupplied in this way, it presents a clear incentive for counterfeiters to fill the unmet demand.
- **Taxes and tariffs.** LDC governments also stimulate

Table 3 Duties and taxes on retail medicines

Country	*Combined total duties and taxes (%)*
India	55
Sierra Leone	40
Nigeria	34
Pakistan	33
Bolivia	32
Bangladesh	29
China	28
Jamaica	27
Morocco	25
Georgia	25
Mexico	24

Source: Adapted from EC (2003)

demand for cheaper fakes by artificially driving up the price of legitimate drugs through taxes and tariffs, which can inflate the retail price of drugs by up to 50% (see Table 3 above). Many of the high-tariff countries also have a significant indigenous counterfeit medicine industry and/or problem. It is unlikely that this is entirely coincidental.

What can be done in Less Developed Countries?

In order to contain the global counterfeiting scourge, it is necessary to address those dynamics which encourage the manufacture and supply of counterfeit medicines. Since the majority of these drugs originate in LDCs, it should be a matter of priority to address those lacunae of governance which allow LDC counterfeiters to ply their trade with relative impunity.

Most importantly, it is essential that contracts, property rights and the rule of law be upheld in the countries where most of these drugs are produced. When properly upheld, these formal market institutions enable entrepreneurs to participate freely in the market, leading to economic growth and technological development. When these institutions are not upheld, as is the case in most lower-income countries, people are forced into the informal economy as a way of sidestepping the cost and difficulty of conducting business formally. And when most of the population subsist within the informal economy, they are unable to avail themselves of the protection that would otherwise exist through contracts or the implied reputation of trademark-protected products.

Some concrete steps to overcome these problems in LDCs include the following:

- Adjudication of disputes over contracts should be simpler and cheaper, so that contracts may be more readily enforced.
- Bureaucratic restrictions on doing business should be removed.
- The manufacturers of brand goods should be able more effectively to protect their trademarks.
- Most fundamentally, courts of law should be granted greater independence, so that their rulings are more impartial and less influenced by powerful vested interests.

- The legislature should not have the power to interfere with judicial decisions.
- The power of law enforcement agents should be curtailed and their actions subject to judicial review.
- The actions of other government agents (e.g. regulators) should be subject to judicial review.
- Regulation restricting the supply of medicines should be improved or scrapped.[15]
- Governments should reduce taxes and tariffs on all medicines.[16]

What can be done internationally?

TRIPs

At the international level, the agreement on trade-related aspects of intellectual property rights (TRIPs), which is part of the WTO Agreements of 1994 and is mandatory for all World Trade Organisation members, requires that the trademark laws of member jurisdictions are compatible with each other, a quality that is known as 'harmonisation'. LDCs that are members of the WTO should therefore have TRIPs-compliant trademark recognition.

The only way for aggrieved countries to police breaches of the TRIPs agreement, however, is through trade sanctions. This is often not a particularly desirable option, for several reasons. First, trade sanctions hurt both parties – people in the offending country will lose much-needed export revenue and associated employment opportunities, while people in the aggrieved country will lose the economic benefits of importing goods from a country that has a comparative advantage in production. To the extent that employment falls in the offending country, more people may end up with a smaller disposable income and thereby are more likely to purchase cheaper counterfeit medicines.

Second, the enforcement of TRIPs can, in certain cases, undermine popular support for intellectual property protection, making future enforcement more difficult politically. For example, in 2001 the research-based pharmaceutical companies sought to challenge in the courts a South African law that seemingly contravened TRIPS. In response to a very vocal campaign by AIDS activists, the pharma companies withdrew their case. While the dispute was not brought in the WTO, the negative PR given to it created a persistent fear of the possible fall-out from bringing such a WTO dispute.

Bilateral trade agreements

An alternative way of persuading LDCs to institute intellectual property regimes is through tempting them with bilateral and regional free trade agreements (FTAs). Most FTAs involving the United States contain provisions that require signatory countries to bolster their intellectual property regimes. By promising access to large and lucrative markets, these agreements can be a way of persuading LDCs to respect the fundamentals of intellectual property protection, which is a vital step towards curtailing counterfeiting.

Although these agreements are not as beneficial as unconditional free trade, they are a step in the right direction, freeing up trade and thereby improving economic well-being. They do, however, raise complications in the form of 'rules of origin' issues, which are costly to monitor and administer. Furthermore, an overly complex 'rules of origin' system may lead to the development of illicit trade routes that could be exploited by traders in illegitimate goods such as counterfeit medicines.

Conclusion

The counterfeiting of drugs is a global problem which will not be eliminated until the supply-side issues are addressed. The majority of counterfeit drugs are manufactured in LDCs, so reform in these countries is absolutely vital if progress is to be made. The most pressing area for reform in most LDCs is the application of the rule of law, the definition and enforceability of property rights and the enforceability of contracts. Without such reforms, counterfeiters will continue to kill hundreds of thousands of people every year.

5

From myth to common wisdom

Graham Satchwell

When I started writing this essay I asked myself, 'Who am I representing? Is it Proco Solutions, the Stockholm Network, the alliance known as "Antidote", my own consultancy or that great new concept, the Healthwell – or indeed the UK Patent Office, or any part of the pharmaceutical industry?' I have specific roles in relation to each of those. They involve representing the public interest, the interests of brand owners, professional colleagues and, of course, me personally. What struck me then was that it does not matter who I 'represent'– the truth is the same, irrespective; for we all have a lot to lose as counterfeiting of medicines becomes more prolific.

There are three main stakeholder groups as far as pharmaceutical safety is concerned. The first is the manufacturer, who always suffers when there is a perceived problem with counterfeiting of their products. No one trusts 'Big Pharma', however, so no one listens to their concerns. Cautionary tales about imported products and the infiltration of counterfeit medicines into the European distribution chain are often seen as Big Pharma's unfair attack on 'Robin Hood parallel traders' motivated by the greed that aggressively protects profit margins. I don't know what sort of a bloke Robin Hood was – he may have been a violent scoundrel with great PR.

I don't know much about history, but I do know that parallel trade is parasitic. Some parasites are good – gut bacteria, for example – some are bad – tics and worms.

The second stakeholder is the person who provides the medicine at the point of final sale, or the person administering the medicine to a member of the public (or patient). These stakeholders have the least control over the distribution network and, as far as the NHS is concerned, are persuaded to buy from the cheapest possible source – not perhaps the most prudent government policy. Yet as 'health professionals', and with media coverage of the problem of counterfeit medicines, they would surely need to defend themselves if they provided counterfeit medicines that caused harm. The question 'Did the pharmacist or doctor take reasonable steps to ensure that counterfeit medicines were not provided?' would quickly arise. Assuming that every product is genuine might well not be regarded as 'reasonable' conduct for much longer.

The third stakeholder, and the most important, is the general public. They remain largely unaware of the true picture.

My message has always been directed at all three groups.

Two years ago I published a book, *Counterfeit Medicines and Organised Crime*, which described the danger of counterfeit medicines entering the legitimate distribution chain in Europe, the inadequacy of the British Medicines and Healthcare Regulatory Agency (MHRA) (under-resourcing and lack of expertise in dealing with crime), and the involvement of organised crime. It was intended as a 'wake-up' call.

It was no great shock to me when the MHRA disowned the implied criticism, refused to acknowledge any weakness or fault in their systems or performance, and assured the public that the distribution chain was safe. Their public statements in 2004 said there was no realistic threat from counterfeit medicines.

Meanwhile the pharmaceutical industry generally remained quiet. The very largest global players employed former senior law enforcement types to investigate on their behalf, most pharmaceutical companies did less, and lots still do very little in that respect – especially the generic manufacturers and the parallel traders.

As I finished writing that book I offered a summary of it free of charge to a young (everyone seems young to me these days) reporter with the *Daily Telegraph*. It seemed to me it would be good for his career and good for the general public. He politely turned it down, explaining that 'I can't create a headline, it's not a simple story', and asking, 'Can you prove how many Britons have died?'

So I thought about how I could best illustrate the weaknesses in our regulatory system and the dangers that the public face, rather than simply describing them in print.

It occurred to me that perhaps I could write a TV documentary outline and convince a national television company to invest in making a documentary …

I decided that when the next big counterfeit medicines incident was reported in the UK, I would immediately conduct my own investigation and illustrate how it is possible to identify the supplier of such medicines very quickly – and then show how the authorities will allow that supplier to continue his dangerous trade for months and months before acting. I knew from painful experience that this was possible. It is invariably the case that wholesalers who are found to have sold counterfeit prescription drugs continue in business, and that they and their suppliers go unnamed for a protracted period, if not indefinitely.

One would reasonably expect that the regulatory enforcement agency would have details of the transactions in question, including, of course, the name of the supplier of the counterfeits, quickly circulated to all UK wholesalers, pharmacists and hospital purchasers. Sadly that is not so.

Why is it not so? I think it is simply because the MHRA has failed to act in a way that suggests their primary duty is to safeguard the public. Can you imagine the outcry if any mainstream investigative agency (say the National Crime Squad or the FBI) always conducted cases in a way that continued to expose individuals to risk of serious injury or death?

At the same time as conducting my own investigation into the counterfeiters I decided to set up in the UK a bogus pharmaceutical wholesale company. I would apply using a false name and get a wholesale dealer's licence from the MHRA and then enter into negotiations with a supplier of counterfeits. In a nutshell I would show how any person bent on making a quick buck could get official authority to deal in prescription medicines and then buy from untrustworthy sources abroad and sell on into the legitimate distribution chain and to the National Health Service.

I wrote that plan in more detail and took it to the executive producer of a very popular British TV documentary series, *Tonight with Trevor McDonald*.

Within weeks I had found premises on an industrial estate in Kent. We paid the rent on a monthly basis. We moved in a PC, a couple of desks, a filing cabinet, a potted plant, a calendar, an answerphone, a fridge (which we rented – in order to pretend that we would, where necessary, store the medicines between certain temperatures, an unnecessary expense!), some cardboard boxes and a few pieces of stationery.

The front company, Oaktree Pharmaceuticals, was never a legal entity, simply a name on the headed paper, a name we spouted when the phone rang, a name we put on the bottom of e-mails, and a name we put on our specially created website.

Two directors were listed. Both names were false, as could have been easily verified. Oaktree Pharmaceuticals was neither a registered company nor a legal partnership nor any other business entity – it was just a name. But nobody checked.

Before anyone can become a wholesale dealer in medicines in the UK they have to appoint a 'responsible person'. This requirement reflects the business reality that those who seek to make money from such products often know nothing about the products or control of stock. The responsible person is therefore important, and is there to ensure that proper records are made of what is purchased, properly stored and dispatched.

One of my colleagues acted as the 'responsible person'. She had previously done this for real, but on this occasion put herself forward using false particulars. But again, no one checked.

A couple of weeks after we had sent off our application to become licensed medicines wholesalers the inspector called by appointment (so no surprise visit that might catch us out). He stayed for about 90 minutes, and his 'inspection' was cursory. We covertly taped it all. No background checks were made on Oaktree Pharmaceuticals, the directors or the responsible person. Let me say that again – no background checks were made on Oaktree Pharmaceuticals, the directors or the responsible person. Ten days later our licence arrived.

As the process of getting that licence continued I returned to the business of drawing in those who were behind the importation of counterfeit Lipitor, which entered the UK legitimate distribution chain in July 2005. For those who don't know, Lipitor is the world's top-selling drug, a life-saver for the many millions who suffer from high cholesterol.

That summer I had spoken to a lot of people in and around the pharmaceutical industry and had a little luck. I very quickly identified the company in the south of England that had bought the stuff from abroad. Unfortunately they had sold it on in some quantity.

Late in July I read an article in *The Times* in which the finding of Lipitor in UK was explained. The article drew heavily on a press release from the MHRA, which said that it was 'thanks to the vigilance of the MHRA' that the counterfeits were found in the United Kingdom. It reassured the British public that the counterfeit Lipitor posed no immediate risk to patients. It seemed to me that the first part of that statement was disingenuous, and the second part dangerous. Yet the press and the public seemed to have accepted the MHRA press release as if it were written on tablets of stone.

The reality was slightly different; the Lipitor matter came to the MHRA's attention because they were warned by customs authorities in Europe that counterfeit Lipitor had been found elsewhere. They, as they are routinely required to do, circulated batch details to wholesalers within the UK in case any had been shipped here. In fact, by no means all wholesalers in UK were advised.

I knew that anyone with knowledge of recent events in the UK (the finding of counterfeit Lipitor, Reductil and Cialis), or who has an awareness of the lack of tight regulatory control here (and elsewhere in Europe), would conclude that the British, like other Europeans, are not properly safeguarded and that the growth in EU membership has merely exacerbated the problem.

It occurred to me then that the US Senate was actively considering whether they should allow the importation of drugs and being reassured by some Europeans that if they did import pharmaceuticals from licensed wholesalers based over here they would have nothing to fear.

In the 'You Americans have nothing to worry about' camp was the UK Medicines and Healthcare Regulatory Authority.

On the MHRA point about counterfeit Lipitor 'posing no immediate risk to patients' it seemed clear to me that medication without the active ingredient, or the wrong active ingredient (in this case the patented Pfizer statin was completely absent from the counterfeits), would result in failure to ameliorate a dangerous condition. Furthermore, if small pharmacies bought sufficient quantities of useless tablets to keep them in stock for six months, and a regular patient was therefore administered a useless product for that period, the condition obviously would not only fail to improve but would worsen. In the case of a dangerously high level of cholesterol the risks were clearly predictable.

In addition, the MHRA press release said nothing about how much of the counterfeit Lipitor might have reached pharmacy shelves or how much of it might be in bathroom cabinets to be consumed by unsuspecting patients in the months ahead. So how much of the counterfeit Lipitor in this case reached patients? No one seemed to have attempted to find out.

And how many other transactions had the UK licensed wholesaler responsible for the counterfeit Lipitor been involved in with this international supplier of counterfeits? No one seems to have bothered to check.

The result of that investigation, and the setting up of my fake business, Oaktree Pharmaceuticals, was televised in the UK in January 2006. I believe the programme does indeed illustrate some of the points that the book describes. I think it is now recognised by some that the book called attention to the extent, nature and dangers of pharmaceutical counterfeiting and parallel trade in a way I believe had not been done before. For too long certain myths have prevailed, and to a dangerous extent they still do.

So what myths prevent governments from taking these matters sufficiently seriously? Why are regulators ill equipped? Why are the press cynical about the issue? Why do the public remain blissfully ignorant? Why are pharmaceutical companies reluctant to speak out?

We must destroy the myths if we are to stop them continuing to destroy lives.

Myth 1: 'Counterfeits are not harmful, they often contain active ingredients'

The underlying assumption here is that counterfeits are some sort of standardised alternative to the real thing. This conclusion is the result of lazy thinking. A few minutes' reflection would mean that people would become aware that of course counterfeits are produced to all sorts of standards, by all sorts of people in all sorts of conditions, in many different countries.

Sometimes production takes place using modern technology (it's worth the investment), sometimes using redundant manufacturing equipment; at other times it is a cottage industry and the product is made by one or many pairs of dirty hands in disgusting conditions. Counterfeit product is never subject to quality testing!

Sometimes the counterfeit will contain more active ingredient than the real thing – which can of course be dangerous. Sometimes there is a like amount, sometimes there is less active ingredient or none – the contents might be entirely inert or poisonous. I say 'inert' rather than harmless, for it is obviously *not* harmless to be taking an inert product when you have a medical condition requiring active treatment.

The truth is: *Counterfeit medicines are always dangerous.*

Myth 2: 'The current concern about counterfeit medicines is just noise made by Big Pharma protecting its profits'

I have no problem with software developers or car manufacturers making a profit, and no problem with pharma companies doing likewise. Unattractive, over-aggressive capitalism, unfettered sufficiently by legal restraint, is unattractive no matter what the product. Every company seeks to maximise profits; it is for the law to fairly restrict them in the public good. But politicians, regulators and commentators who turn away from the danger that the public faces, who smirk and say 'Show me the bodies', make it easy for counterfeits to continue to enter our systems. 'Show us the bodies' could yet prove not simply cynical; it may well prove a disastrous and prophetic injunction.

In Europe we have individuals who buy medicines at cheaper prices in poorer parts of the Continent and repack them so that they display the language of the country in which they will be resold. This happens not only with medicines but with many different sorts of goods – jeans, wine, cigarettes, soft drinks, toothpaste, etc. Now we consumers share the benefit, we buy a (parallel-traded) product here more cheaply, and the importer (the parallel trader) takes a cut. All is well and good. You don't need to repack jeans, however; they cannot be worn unsafely or stored in a manner that disrupts their efficacy! It does not matter too much if a 32-inch waist is shown as a 34-inch; you can try them on before buying. Not so with medicines, though; discovering you have the wrong dosage, or that the information leaflet is useless, is rather more intimidating.

So who makes the profit from parallel trade? The parallel traders, who provide us all with cheaper goods – but when it comes to pharmaceuticals they need to be properly regulated, inspected and monitored. There is no logical reason why the safety of medicines should be compromised so that middlemen can make an extra buck.

The truth is: *Parallel trade in medicines is parasitic; only sometimes does the host benefit.*

Myth 3: 'Counterfeits are a Third World issue; there have been no significant cases in the Western world'

Needless thousands die every year as a direct consequence of taking counterfeit medicines; yes, they are Chinese, Asian and African. But these are not racist crimes – there is no reason to think that the manufacturers of counterfeit product care more about European or American lives than, say, Korean lives – in fact the opposite might well be true. It has been over two years since my book warned that deaths obviously linked to this trade would occur in the West – now sadly they have, but those Canadian deaths will not be an isolated tragedy. All trade is now global, thanks mostly to the Internet. Products that once caused death only in China and Africa are now advertised as available for sale in Europe. It would be stupid to think that those foreigners capable of killing their own countrymen would not sell deadly medicines to us. And it would be equally stupid to think that Western criminals will not take advantage of the opportunity to buy such products and sell them into the most lucrative markets in the world – the USA, the UK, Germany, France and the like.

It has been two years since that book warned that counterfeit medicines would be identified as having entered the legitimate distribution chain – since which time they have, more than once.

The truth is: *Counterfeit medicines pose a real danger to both developed and developing countries.*

Myth 4: 'In any case, pharma companies put holograms on their packs, so you can tell by this and the other aspects of the high-quality packaging on the real thing'

The truth is that anyone, pharmacist or consumer, who thinks that the presence of a hologram is surety enough is a fool. It is true to say that pharmaceutical companies should know, if they don't, and many certainly do, that some of the counterfeit holograms are more convincing than the real thing. For the record, it takes about two weeks to have a 'new' hologram copied. And by the way, show me a person who says they can tell a counterfeit from looking at the medication or the pack and I'll show you a fool.

There are much better systems for protecting the supply chain than holograms and 'micro text' – but the pharmaceutical industry has yet to come to terms with the need to increase costs to provide adequate security in the supply chain. In addition, such anti-counterfeiting packaging features are rendered useless when packaging is entirely removed to facilitate parallel trade repackaging.

In the USA medicines are commonly provided loose in plastic or glass bottles; Americans would be impressed by European packaging standards (if it is possible for Americans to be impressed by anything European these days). How can the wealthiest country in the world tolerate medicinal packaging conventions that are miles behind those of Europe?

In the last few months one or two major manufacturers have started RFID-tagging certain products. It is time that the pace of change quickened and that each party in the distribution chain, manufacturer, distributor, wholesaler, pharmacist, and consumer, had the means to verify the authenticity of the medicines in front of them.

The truth is: *You can't tell a counterfeit medicine from the real thing until it's too late.*

Myth 5: 'Customs and other regulators have systems to stop counterfeits being imported'

This is one of the most dangerous myths. It implies that Britons, Germans and Americans are all cosy and safe because of the border controls in place. The truth is that the British and Germans long ago largely ceded their borders to wider European border protection, and that is no better than the worst-performing southern or eastern European border agency. Of course, we still have a domestic customs service, as do many others within Europe. But check with your customs authorities – it is impossible for customs and postal services to monitor the contents of the billions of tonnes of imports into the UK or anywhere else in Europe. What percentage of containers bringing imported goods into our country is opened and checked? Less than 3%. Something like 97% passes without examination. That's a very low risk of detection, and well worth a dishonest bet.

And when customs authorities in the UK find small quantities of pharmaceuticals, prescribed medicines, going to non-registered dealers, what do they do? They charge them VAT and send the package on!

The truth is: *Most imported goods, whether bulk import by container or by post, are not examined on entering the country.*

Myth 6: 'If I don't buy off the Internet and only get my prescriptions filled at regular pharmacists, or take drugs provided while in hospital, then I will be safe'

It is amazing that intelligent people still believe that counterfeit medicines are something that the naive and desperate buy cheaply over the Internet or elsewhere. And that if you avoid the Internet you can avoid fake drugs. The reality is that the opportunities to buy direct from the Net are taken not only by fools, but also by unscrupulous Western dealers who are quite happy to import and sell on to unsuspecting pharmacists, wholesalers who then supply hospitals and high-street pharmacies.

The truth is: *Wherever you get medicines from you cannot be sure of their origin or whether they are not counterfeit; your doctor or pharmacist can be fooled as easily as you.*

Myth 7: 'Talk of involvement of organised crime is just scare-mongering'

This is a variation on the 'Big Pharma noise' myth described in Myth 2. The involvement of organised crime can be confirmed in two ways, the first employing pure logic. Why would organised crime not get involved in a multi-million-pound crime that is so easy to commit, which provides such anonymity and such huge profits, generates such little interest on the part of law enforcement agencies, thereby invariably going unnoticed, and which is part of a growth industry?

The second involves not logic but clear evidence of two types – direct evidence of actual cases and expert opinion.

If you want cases (for example, involving the Camorra, the Florida cases, any of the many Chinese cases, or details of the multiple deaths in Nigeria), then refer to my book *A Sick Business. Counterfeit Medicines and Organised Crime.*[1] Or do some research with Interpol or the FDA or NASDAQ or the Chinese authorities or the UK National Criminal Intelligence Service.

Expert opinion? Try the head of Interpol, the head of the British National Criminal Intelligence Service, umpteen FBI people, and many experienced investigators.

The fact is that while there are vast amounts of money to be made out of this illegal death-causing trade it is inconceivable that organised crime should not be involved.

The truth is: *With all the money to be made, an expanding and gullible market, the low risk of detection, and ease of operation, it would be really silly if organised crime were not seriously involved.*

Myth 8: 'If drugs are offered for sale from Spain or France or Ireland or the UK then they must be OK'

In the last twelve months within the UK we have discovered three separate cases of counterfeit medicines entering the legitimate chain, involving Reductil, Cialis and Lipitor. We did not find them as a result of the UK's monitoring or intelligence system. In the UK the regulatory authority is not particularly well resourced or, I might add, particularly effective; much more worryingly, it is one of the better European healthcare regulatory agencies.

It has been revealed in the last few weeks (at a conference in Rome) that Europe has seen many drugs-counterfeiting incidents that have not previously been made public. The very porous borders of eastern Europe provide further opportunities for unscrupulous businessmen on both sides of the border. Those opportunities are unlikely to pass unnoticed. Unless we are to have our poorly regulated systems taken advantage of to an even greater extent, then we need to motivate all stakeholders to greater action.

Any reliance placed upon the distribution systems in Europe to vouchsafe imports to the USA is badly misplaced.

European regulatory agencies are vital public bodies charged with a responsibility to protect the public from exposure to potentially lethal counterfeit medicines. The knock-on effect of that role is that they also serve the interests of pharmacists, wholesalers, parallel importers and manufacturers. No legitimate business benefits from the presence of counterfeit pharmaceuticals in the legitimate market; each is potentially legally liable and each can suffer damage to reputation and consequent business loss. The effectiveness of the regulatory agencies is important to us all.

Many questions about the European regulatory agencies remain unanswered here. For instance, what do manufacturers privately say about liaison with such agencies? What do parallel traders think of the amount of supervision and inspection they are subjected to? Are current repackaging regulations and inspections adequate? How concerned are pharmacists when regulators descend on them? How hard can regulatory agencies hit organised crime? Are the staff of such agencies trained in conducting major investigations? Can they put a team of investigators and crime analysts together under a senior investigating officer to conduct a major investigation in the way one would expect of any police force?

Traditionally medicines regulatory bodies have had no need to be resourced for or skilled in collation and analysis of criminal intelligence, in setting up major crime investigations or managing covert investigations, handling confidential informants or deploying undercover staff.

It may be that many European medicines regulatory bodies do not see it as their role to undertake such activities or to facilitate them.

In the event of a catastrophic incidence of deaths from counterfeiting (and who would now say it could not occur?), such agencies may yet just 'wash their hands' of any responsibility and rely on the claim that 'It is not our role to investigate major crime.'

There have been hints in the past that they see themselves

merely as 'regulatory' agencies and not 'crime investigation' agencies. This would suggest that their role is to license, inspect and bring to book, where necessary, those responsible for non-compliance with regulations concerning the conduct of lawful business. This position differentiates breach of regulation from breach of the criminal law. In the UK, for example, the MHRA has no power to bring charges under anything other than its regulatory legislation. The agency cannot prosecute for counterfeiting, fraud or manslaughter, so the 'fall-back' defence is ready and could be used to quickly move ownership of a catastrophe to the police.

If that is the fall-back position the MHRA would seek, then ownership of the problem needs to pass immediately to the police and the police service needs to get more involved on the intelligence side on a regular basis without delay.

Currently the US government is considering whether to allow the importation of drugs. Before European authorities can be perfectly honest in advising the US authorities on the potential dangers from imported counterfeit medicine they will need to be more open and honest with the British public. When that happens then greater reliance will be placed on the cautionary tales being told by 'Big Pharma', myths will be exploded and pharmacists and health professionals will have a heightened awareness of the problems. The general public, on both sides of the Atlantic, will then be much better served.

Notes

Chapter 1 Counterfeit medicines and pharmaceutical crime in Europe

1. CEP (also known as CoS) is the Certificate of Suitability of European Pharmacopoeia monographs and is intended to demonstrate that the purity of a given substance produced by a given manufacturer is suitability-controlled by the relevant monograph(s) of the European Pharmacopoeia.
2. The proposed directive supplements Directive 2004/48/EC of 29 April 2004 on the enforcement of intellectual property rights.
3. The WHO counterfeit medicine database system is not used satisfactorily by many European states. Perhaps part of the reason for this is that the database is not linked to any direct regulatory responsive action.
4. A move towards more European centralisation of MA procedures.
5. 'Future of Europol. Is Europol becoming a European FBI?', www.ex.ac.uk/~watupman/undergrad/pollard/html/future.htm.

6. A significant initial attempt at codification and cross-referencing of potentially applicable European and state level legislation was made as part of the CoE survey analysis, but was not finally included in the report as the available data received were not entirely complete.
7. For example, an Internet pharmacy verification system (the US system may provide a model for Europe).
8. Existing API monographs require updating and made more complete (in order to permit effective analytical testing) and internationally harmonised; the ICH Q7A GMP API guideline requires full adoption and implementation in the EU.

Chapter 3 Finding common ground: policy imperatives for Europe

1. This chapter sets out the central policy direction and associated actions needed to thwart the trade in counterfeit prescription medicines. It was originally presented at the Washington conference on counterfeiting in September 2005, and revised for a European audience in Brussels in February 2006.
2. We have some knowledge from current inadequate surveillance and sporadic journalistic reporting that counterfeit drugs are already a risk in some parts of Africa and Asia, with fake drugs now appearing in other parts of the world with serious, if not fatal, consequences for human health (Cockburn et al., 2005).
3. 'Hamilton pharmacist charged with handing out counterfeit drugs', CBC, 10 September 2005, accessed at www.cbc.

ca/story/science/national/2005/09/10/counterfeit_
drugs20050910.html.

4. This work was undertaken for the UK pharmaceutical industry, but does not represent the position of the Association of the British Pharmaceutical Industry. Additional material on the safety chain is available from the author or at www.policyinsider.com.

5. Primarily Directive 2001/83/EC of the European Parliament and of the Council of 6 November 2001 on the Community code relating to medicinal products for human use. See also Directive 2004/27/EC of the European Parliament and of the Council of 31 March 2004 amending Directive 2001/83/EC on the Community code relating to medicinal products for human use. Available at www.pharmacos.eudra.org/f2/eudralex/vol-1/home.htm.

6. Article 152, Treaty of Rome, 7 February 1957 (consolidated version).

7. European Commission, *Commission Communication on parallel imports of proprietary medicinal products for which marketing authorisations have already been granted*, COM(2003)839; and also European Commission, *The Internal Market and Health Services: Report of the High Level Committee on Health*, 17 December 2001.

8. COM(2003)839, §5.5, note 45.

9. Patient safety has featured as a top priority of the Luxembourg and UK presidencies and this dossier continues to be carried forward; *The Luxembourg Declaration on Patient Safety*, 5 April 2005.

10. Council Directive 92/28/EEC of 31 March 1992 on the advertising of medicinal products for human use.
11. See Harper, this volume.
12. Adapted from *Integrated Public Safety Policy*, Ministry of the Interior, Government of the Netherlands, 1993.
13. International Maritime Organisation, *ISM Code (International Safety Management Code) and revised guidelines on implementation of the ISM Code* (IMO-IA117E), 2002 edn.
14. Food Safety Act 1990, §21.

Chapter 4 Counterfeit medicines in less developed countries

1. www.who.int/mediacentre/factsheets/fs275/en/.
2. European Federation of Pharmaceutical Industries and Associations, 'Counterfeit medicines', available at www.efpia.org/2_indust/counterfeitdrugs.pdf.
3. www.manilatimes.net/national/2005/aug/16/yehey/life/20050816lif1.html.
4. http://bmj.bmjjournals.com/cgi/content/full/327/7424/1126-a.
5. www.who.int/entity/bulletin/volumes/81/12/WHONews.pdf.
6. http://bmj.bmjjournals.com/cgi/content/full/327/7412/414-b.
7. http://pharmalicensing.com/articles/disp/1120475327_42c918bf09048.

8. 'Selling cheap generic drugs, India's copycats irk industry', available at http://chakra.org/articles/2000/12/03/indian/drugs.

9. 'Latin America battles counterfeit drug threat, daily international pharmacy alert', *Washington Business Information*, 2(292), 2006.

10. www.efpia.org/2_indust/counterfeitdrugs.pdf.

11. 'Fake drugs worry authorities, firms', *Russia Journal*, 3(4): 47.

12. *South China Business Journal*, June/July/August 2002.

13. www.prospect.org/web/page.ww?section=root&name=ViewWeb&articleId=10650.

14. www.freemarketfoundation.com/ShowArticle.asp?ArticleType=Publication&ArticleID=1093.

15. Very often, the supply of drugs is reduced by the byzantine and tortuous regulations that emanate from local drug approval agencies. These regulations make it very difficult for manufacturers wishing to export to overseas markets to register new products, thereby creating a gap in supply. This gap provides another opportunity for counterfeiters.

16. These artificial price inflators can price many patients out of treatment, and give them an incentive to look to cheaper counterfeit medicines to meet their needs. Abolishing these levies would return medicines to their natural prices, thereby undermining the potential profits – and incentives – of counterfeiters.

Chapter 5 From myth to common wisdom

1. Stockholm Network, London, 2004.

References

Chapter 1 Counterfeit medicines and pharmaceutical crime in Europe

BBC News (2006), 'Agency to target brutal crime', 3 April 2006, http://news.bbc.co.uk/1/hi/uk/4870988.stm.

CEIPI (2004), 'Impacts de la contrefaçon et de la piraterie en Europe, rapport final', Centre d'Etudes Internationales de la Propriété Industrielle, 9 July.

CoE (2004), *Counterfeiting: Problems and Solutions*, Recommendation 1673, Parliamentary Assembly, Council of Europe.

EC (2005), 'Proposal for a European Parliament and Council Directive on criminal measures aimed at ensuring the enforcement of intellectual property rights', COM(2005)276 final 2005/0127(COD) 2005/0128(CNS), Brussels: European Commission, 12 July.

EC (2006), 'Commission warns about fake drugs on the internet', Brussels: European Commission, 27 March, http://europa.eu.int/rapid/pressReleasesAction.do?reference=IP/06/375&type=%20HTML&aged=0&language=EN&guiLanguage=en.

FDA (2001), 'Frances Oldham Kelsey: FDA medical reviewer leaves her mark on history', *FDA Consumer Magazine*, March/April, www.fda.gov/FDAC/features/2001/201_kelsey.html.

FDA (2004), *Verified Internet Pharmacy Practice Sites (VIPPS)*, Washington, DC: Food and Drugs Administration, www.fda.gov/cder/consumerinfo/counterfeitdrugsLo.pdf.

Harper, J. R. (2006), *Counterfeit Medicines Survey Report. Harmonised Provisions for Legislative and Administrative Procedures applicable to Counterfeit Medicines in the Council of Europe Member States*, Strasbourg: Council of Europe Publishing.

IGZ (Netherlands Health Care Inspectorate) (2005), 'More stringent checks required from pharmaceuticals distributors for counterfeit pharmaceutical drugs and supplier and customer authorisation', October.

Kanavos, P. et al. (2004), 'The economic impact of pharmaceutical parallel trade in European Union member states: a stakeholder analysis', London: LSE; January, www.lse.ac.uk/collections/LSEHealthAndSocialCare/pdf/Workingpapers/Paper.pdf.

Newton-Dunn, B. (2004), 'Europe needs an FBI', September, www.publicaffairs.ac/articles/EuropeanFBI.pdf.

O'Mathuna, D. P. and A. McAuley (2005), *Counterfeit Drugs: Towards an Irish Response to a Global Crisis*, Dublin: Irish Patients Association.

Republic of the Philippines (2003), 'An Act prohibiting drugs, providing penalties for violations and appropriating funds therefor', No. 8203.

Satchwell, G. (2004), *A Sick Business. Counterfeit Medicines and Organised Crime*, London: Stockholm Network.

Single Convention on Narcotic Drugs (1961), as amended by the 1972 Protocol Amending the Single Convention on Narcotic Drugs, 1961; Convention on Psychotropic Substances 1971 Including Final Act and Resolutions, as agreed by the 1971

United Nations Conference for the Adoption of a Protocol on Psychotropic Substances, and the Schedules annexed to the Convention; United Nations Convention Against Illicit Traffic in Narcotic Drugs and Psychotropic Substances, 1988 Including Final Act and Resolutions, as agreed by the United Nations Conference for the Adoption of a Convention against Illicit Traffic in Narcotic Drugs and Psychotropic Substances, and the Tables annexed to the Convention.

Wesch, M. W. (2004), 'Strafbarkeit von Arzneimittelfalschern', *Pharm. Ind.*, 66(7): 872–73.

WHO (2006a) *Counterfeit Medicines*, WHO fact sheet no. 275, revised February, www.who.int/mediacentre/factsheets/fs275/en.

WHO (2006b), *Declaration of Rome*, WHO International Conference on 'Combating counterfeit drugs: building effective international collaboration', Rome, 18 February.

Chapter 2 Facing the reality of medicines counterfeiting

Anderson, M. (2006), Personal communication.

Behrnt, N. (2006), 'Combat counterfeit medicines – views from a regional organisation (EU)', WHO conference, Rome, 16–18 February.

Carlton (2006), *Tonight* programme transcript, 9 January.

EFPIA (2006), www.efpia.org, last accessed 26 March 2006.

Haines, A. (2006), Personal communication.

Harper, J. R. (2006), *Counterfeit Medicines Survey Report. Harmonised Provisions for Legislative and Administrative Procedures applicable to Counterfeit Medicines in the Council of Europe Member States*, Strasbourg: Council of Europe Publishing.

Kanavos, P., D. Gross and D. Taylor (2005), *Parallel Trading in Medicines. Europe's experience and its implications for commercial drug importation in the US*, Washington, DC: American Association for Retired Persons.

O'Mathuna, D. P. and A. McAuley (2005), *Counterfeit Drugs: Towards an Irish Response to a Global Crisis*, Dublin: Irish Patients Association.

Satchwell, G. (2004). *A Sick Business. Counterfeit Medicines and Organised Crime*, London: Stockholm Network.

Taylor, D., M. Mrazek and E. Mossialos (2004), 'Regulating pharmaceutical distribution and retail pharmacy in Europe', in Mossialos, Mrazek and Whalley (eds), *Regulating the Cost and Use of Pharmaceuticals in Europe*, Copenhagen: WHO Europe.

Transparency International (2006), *Global Corruption Report 2006: Corruption and Health*, London: Pluto Press.

Chapter 3 Finding common ground: policy imperatives for Europe

Cockburn, R., P. Newton, E. K. Agyarko, D. Akunyili and N. White (2005), 'The global threat of counterfeit drugs: why industry and governments must communicate the dangers', *PLoS Medicine*, 2(4): e100.

Eban, K. (2005), *Dangerous Dose: How counterfeiters are contaminating America's drug supply*, New York: Harcourt.

IoM (Institute of Medicine) (2000),*To Err Is Human*, Washington, DC: National Academy Press.

Rittel, H. J. (1972), 'Second generation design methods', Interview in Design Methods Group 5th Anniversary Report, DMG Occasional Paper no. 1, pp. 5–10.

Rittel, H. J. and M. M. Webber (1973), 'Dilemmas in a general theory of planning', *Policy Sciences*, 4: 155–69.

Rittel, H. J. and M. M. Webber (1984), 'Planning problems are wicked problems', in N. Cross (ed.), *Developments in Design Methodology*, Chichester: Wiley, pp. 135–44.

Satchwell, G. (2004), *A Sick Business. Counterfeit Medicines and Organised Crime*, London: Stockholm Network.

Tickner, J., C. Raffensperger and N. Myers (1998), *The Precautionary Principle in Action: a Handbook*, Science and Environmental Health Network.

Walshe, K. (2003), *Regulating Healthcare: a Prescription for Improvement*, Milton Keynes: Open University Press.

WHO (2006), *Declaration of Rome*, WHO International Conference on 'Combating counterfeit drugs: building effective international collaboration', Rome, 18 February.

Chapter 4 Counterfeit medicines in less developed countries

Ahmad, K. (2004), 'Antidepressants are sold as antiretrovirals in DR Congo', *The Lancet*, 363: 713.

Cockburn, R., P. Newton, E. K. Agyarko, D. Akunyili and N. White (2005), 'The global threat of counterfeit drugs: why industry and governments must communicate the dangers', *PLoS Medicine*, 2(4): e100

Dondorp, A., P. Newton, M. Mayxay, W. van Damme, F. Smithuis, S. Yeung, A. Petit, A. Lynam, A. Johnson, T. Hien, R. McGready, J. Farrar, S. Looareesuwan, N. Day, M. Green and N. White (2004), 'Fake antimalarials in Southeast Asia are a major impediment to malaria control: multinational cross-sectional survey on the prevalence of fake antimalarials', *Tropical Medicine & International Health*, 9(12): 1241.

EC (2003), 'Working document on developing countries' duties and taxes on essential medicines used in the treatment of major communicable diseases', Brussels: European Commission, Directorate-General for Trade.

Fackler, M (2002), 'China's fake drugs kill thousands', *San Francisco Examiner*, 29 July.

Gibson, L. (2004), 'Drug regulators study global treaty to tackle counterfeit drugs', *British Medical Journal*, 328(486).

Hanif, M., M. Mobarak, A. Ronan, D. Rahman, J. Donovan et al. (1995), 'Fatal renal failure caused by diethylene glycol in paracetamol elixir: the Bangladesh epidemic', *British Medical Journal*, 311: 88–91.

Pécoul, B., P. Chirac, P. Trouiller, J. Pine (1999), 'Access to essential drugs in poor countries – a lost battle?', *JAMA*, 281(4).

Raufu, A. (2003), 'India agrees to help Nigeria tackle the import of fake drugs', *British Medical Journal*, 326: 1234.

Shakoor, O., R. Taylor, R. Behrens (1997), 'Assessment of the incidence of substandard drugs in developing countries', *Tropical Medicine & International Health*, 2(9): 839–45.

White, N. (1999), 'Delaying antimalarial drug resistance with combination chemotherapy', *Parassitologia*, 41: 301–308.

WHO (2003), 'The quality of antimalarials: a study in seven African countries', Geneva: WHO, available at http://whqlibdoc.who.int/hq/2003/WHO_EDM_PAR_2003.4.pdf.

Joining the Stockholm Network

Would you or your organisation like to join the Stockholm Network? We have varying levels of membership, depending on your needs and interests. For further information, please contact our Director of Development, Nicole Gray Conchar (nicole@stockholm-network.org).

Subscribe to the mailing list

Fancy getting a taste of what we do and what think tanks are doing right across Europe? The Stockholm Network's weekly e-newsletter rounds up the latest activities of Europe's leading think tanks and thinkers and provides a valuable summary of current policy trends across the EU. To sign up, contact Sacha James Kumaria (sacha@stockholm-network.org), or visit our website: www.stockholm-network.org.

Other titles recently published by the Stockholm Network are listed on the following pages

Impatient for Change

European attitudes to healthcare reform

Helen Disney, Karen Horn, Pavel Hrobon, Johan Hjertqvist, Alastair Kilmarnock, Andreas Mihm, Alberto Mingardi, Cécile Philippe, David Smith, Eline van den Broek, Gerrold Verhoeks

Do Europe's politicians really understand what voters want from their healthcare systems? How can they square the circle of rising demand, rising costs and shrinking tax funding?

To find out, the Stockholm Network and Populus commissioned a major study of the European public's attitudes on the state of their health systems now and what they expect from them in future. Leading healthcare experts from across Europe analyse the data, putting it into its national and pan-European context.

The results are startling. Europeans are becoming ever more concerned about what will happen to their health provision in future if reform is not carried out urgently. They demonstrate a large gap between what patients want and what their political elite is delivering. And they suggest that information and gaining the support of the medical profession are crucial to securing the reform that Europe's ailing health systems need. Europe's health consumers are already waiting and impatient for change.

Published in association with Populus
ISBN: 0-9547663-0-X
£12.00

An Apology for Capitalism?

Matthew Bishop, Vincent Cable, Clive Crook, Howard Davies, Bill Durodié, Stephen Godfrey-Isaacs, Julia Hailes, David Henderson, Steve Hilton, Benjamin Hunt, John Kay, Philippe Legrain, Johan Norberg, Neil Sherlock, Stephen Tindale

Edited by Helen Disney

Should companies be cheerleaders for capitalism or is the growth of corporate and social responsibility evidence of a new way of doing business and doing it better? Is it time for policy-makers and business leaders to be more aggressive in dealing with business failure?

A backlash is emerging too among those who think companies are becoming too timid and apologetic. Too much of this risk aversion could be damaging not just to profits but to faith in capitalism itself. With books critical of global corporations topping best-seller lists across the world, how can corporations answer their critics – and should they even try?

An Apology for Capitalism? assembles leading thinkers and policy experts to debate the limits of corporate and social responsibility. It questions whether corporations deserve the flak and asks if it is now time for them to embrace the business of saying sorry.

ISBN: 0-9547663-1-8
£10.00

A Sick Business

Counterfeit medicines and organised crime

Graham Satchwell

Foreword by Lord Mackenzie of Framwellgate

Conducted by a former policeman, this investigation into the trade in fake medicines and its links with organised crime uncovers a horrifying story. Across Europe, counterfeiters have discovered a range of easy routes for selling fake and sub-standard products into the legitimate distribution chain.

A Sick Business shows how, to the uninitiated eye, this crime is invisible. Most patients and consumers are unaware of just how many public safety problems counterfeit medicines may cause. It reveals that this illegal business is conducted by unscrupulous people whose actions have already cost thousands of lives and may even be linked to terrorist activity – yet almost nothing is being done to stop it.

It should be read by anyone with an interest in keeping Europe safe.

ISBN 0-9547663-2-6
£10.00

Poles Apart?

Eastern European attitudes to healthcare reform

Helen Disney, David Hill, Pavel Hrobon, Adam Kruszewski, Henrieta Madarová, Rick Nye, Martin Stefunko

How have eastern European countries fared since the fall of the Berlin Wall, and what do their attitudes tell us about the prospects for healthcare reform today?

Poles Apart? sets out to examine whether the perception of a superior western European healthcare system is really true by asking the opinions of 3,000 central and eastern Europeans and comparing them with their counterparts in the rest of the EU.

Despite differences in access to care, due to significantly lower levels of funding, and a sometimes unfounded admiration of western Europe, the challenges facing healthcare systems and the way people view them are remarkably similar across the board. More striking still, the new Europe's attitude suggests that the east is on the cusp of providing valuable inspiration and experience for reformers in western Europe in shaping the modern health systems of tomorrow.

Published in association with Populus
ISBN: 0-9547663-3-4
£10.00

Does the West Know Best?

Martin Bruncko, Gabriel Calzada, Christofer Fjellner, Andrei Grecu, Johan Hjertqvist, Pavel Hrobon, Philippe Manière, Miroslav Mikolasik, Dan Mitchell, Johnny Munkhammar, Stephen O'Connor, Matus Petrik, Ugnius Trumpa

Edited by Terence O'Dwyer

Accession of the central and eastern European states has provided impetus for a fundamental re-evaluation of Europe's economic and social model. New member states have challenged the orthodoxy of western European systems. With the west now facing the impending crises of an aging population and unsustainable healthcare systems, and the prospect of sustained weak economic growth, the questions are: Should the new member states be emulating western Europe? Or should 'old Europe' mimic the reforms of its newest partners? Indeed, does 'old Europe' have any choice but to reform?

Does the West Know Best? assembles leading European thinkers to examine social and economic reform, such as flat taxation, the privatisation of social security and moves towards more market-oriented health systems. It questions the sustainability of the European economic and social model, while seeking solutions to its endemic problems.

ISBN: 0-9547663-4-2

£8.00

Intellectual Property Frontiers

Expanding the borders of discussion

Edited by Dr Meir Pugatch and Anne K. Jensen

The first book to be published by the Stockholm Network's Intellectual Property and Competition programme, *Intellectual Property Frontiers* draws on the expertise of eighteen distinguished scholars, policymakers and practitioners. It aims to familiarise readers with the diversity of themes and debates currently taking place in the field of IP.

The publication is divided into four sections:

- The role of intellectual property in the business arena;
- Intellectual property dilemmas;
- Global issues;
- The European perspective.

£8.00

Europe Needs Saving

Defusing the pensions timebomb

Matthew Bishop, Liam Halligan, Kamil Kajetanowicz, Edward Palmer, Giuseppe Pennisi, Wilfried Prewo, L. Jacobo Rodríguez, Ian Vásquez

Edited by Terence O'Dwyer

We are facing a demographic time bomb: by 2050, there will be two workers to every retired person in most European countries. In some countries, that ratio will be 1:1. Current pay-as-you-go pension systems are quite simply financially, economically and socially unsustainable – without reform, pensioners will bankrupt the welfare state.

In *Europe Needs Saving,* several internationally renowned experts on pensions attempt to answer some of the most difficult questions facing us today: Should pay-as-you-go systems be tweaked only slightly? Is there a role for the market in providing pensions? If so, how extensive should that role be? What are the benefits to the citizen – and to the government? What can be learned from countries that have already reformed? Is the Chilean model suitable for the ailing systems in Europe? Or is the Swedish approach to reform more appropriate?

ISBN-10: 0-9547663-7-7
ISBN-13: 978-0-9547663-7-5
£10.00